# Psychoanalytic Psychotherapy in Psychiatric Practice

In this uniquely intimate and clinical book, Mark Kinet explores the vital role of psychodynamic psychotherapy in psychiatric work.

*Psychoanalytic Psychotherapy in Psychiatric Practice: Premises and Clinical Portraits* includes over 70 case studies of patients receiving psychiatric care in various settings, from (semi-)residential treatment to outpatient support. Kinet draws on his extensive experience of conducting group and individual psychotherapy sessions, psychoanalysis in a traditional setting, and his integration of play therapy techniques. He introduces and explores seven foundational premises essential to the success of psychodynamic psychotherapy with these patients: the integration of intrapsychic and interpersonal forces and perspectives, the key impact of unconscious content and processes, the vital importance of the therapeutic relationship, the mobilisation of mentalising capacities, the interpretation of hidden motives, the emancipation resulting from enlightenment, and the importance of approaching this work with realism rather than an idealised perspective. The case studies highlight common mental issues such as anxiety, low mood and clinical depression, PTSD, and personality disorders, equipping the reader with the tools to understand and help a wide range of patients.

Written in accessible language, this volume will be of great interest to psychiatrists, psychoanalysts, and psychotherapists, as well as anyone interested in gaining insight into real-life psychiatric practice.

**Mark Kinet** is a psychiatrist, psychotherapist, and psychoanalyst based in Belgium. He is the author of *The Spirit of the Drive in Neuropsychoanalysis* (2023) and *Psychoanalytic Principles in Psychiatric Practice. A Remedy by Truth* (2024).

"With over thirty years of impressive experience in full-time clinical work, the author is a trusted figure in the field. He is an integrative and independent psychiatrist and psychoanalyst, taking an autonomous stance towards the various psychoanalytic schools. His unique perspective is abundantly illustrated in 77 portraits or case studies. This book is a relevant and valuable resource for all those involved in mental health care: patients, therapists, counsellors, medical doctors, nurses ... You must read this book!"

**Marc Hebbrecht, M.D.**, psychiatrist, IPA psychoanalyst, current president of the Belgian Society of Psychoanalysis and the former editor-in-chief of *Tijdschrift voor Psychoanalyse* (Dutch Journal of Psychoanalysis)

"Although structured differently, this is a kind of 'companion book' to Kinet's *Psychoanalytic Principles in Psychiatric Practice*. A brief outline of seven premises is followed by 77 concise case histories presented in straightforward terms. These mainly deal with severe psychiatric problems, which are, or instead appear to be, workable on a psychoanalytic basis. That this turns out to be possible in our time of 'disorder-centred treatment modules', is surprising and hopeful – for current psychiatry and for current psychoanalysis. So this is how it can be done! The clinical data are captivatingly described and get to the heart of the matter quickly, inviting the reader's thinking."

**Antoine Mooij, M.D., PhD**, psychiatrist, psychoanalyst, philosopher, emeritus professor at the University of Utrecht (NL), Netherlands

"In this highly readable book, psychoanalytic therapist and clinical psychiatrist Mark Kinet reflects on the power and practice of contemporary psychotherapy. Uniquely, he opens up the lives of 77 former patients, allowing the reader to see the challenges patients and therapists face. As a series, these case studies clarify what abstract psychodynamic concepts like transference, mentalisation, or interpretation imply – or might imply – in clinical practice."

**Stijn Vanheule, PhD**, clinical psychologist, professor of psychoanalysis and clinical psychology at the University of Gent (B), Belgium

"This book gives us a direct and thoughtful insight into what psychoanalytic practice in its diverse forms implies. It consistently builds further on the earlier volume of Mark Kinet's trilogy on psychoanalysis in all its clinical and psychiatric applications. Indeed, we are far from the illusion of a monolithic and dogmatic doctrine under the direction of primal father Sigmund Freud (and/or Jacques Lacan). The many, sharply written, short case studies demonstrate the multifaceted nature of the psychoanalytical approach. The common thread is the ethics of psychoanalysis: the fundamental respect for every human person – their history, choices, preferences, inclinations, etc. – and the dialogical effort to promote the liberation of the person from what hinders their personal development and prevents growth."

**Jozef Corveleyn**, clinical psychologist, psychoanalyst and emeritus professor at KULeuven (B), Belgium

"Over thirty years of clinical experience in psychoanalytic psychotherapy leaps off the pages. The author speaks as a psychiatrist who genuinely enjoys his profession, skilfully applying psychoanalytic thinking in both clinical and (semi)residential settings. With its accessible language, the text allows readers unfamiliar with the field to empathise with the client and their journey, while colleagues will appreciate the refreshingly unorthodox approach."

**Frans Schalkwijk**, psychoanalyst in private practice, former editor-in-chief of *Tijdschrift voor Psychoanalyse* (Dutch Journal of Psychoanalysis), and emeritus professor at the University of Amsterdam (NL), Netherlands

# Psychoanalytic Psychotherapy in Psychiatric Practice

Premises and Clinical Portraits

Mark Kinet

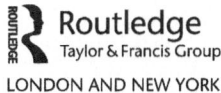
Routledge
Taylor & Francis Group

LONDON AND NEW YORK

First Dutch edition published by Gompel&Svacina 2018
First English edition published by Routledge 2025

ISBN: 978-1-032-79126-5 (hbk)
ISBN: 978-1-032-74331-8 (pbk)
ISBN: 978-1-003-49060-9 (ebk)

DOI: 10.4324/9781003490609

Typeset in Times New Roman
by Taylor & Francis Books

*Non ignora mali, miseris succurrere disco.*
Not ignorant of bad things, I learn to help the wretched.
(Dixit Dido in Virgil's Aeneid, 1.630)

# Contents

1   Prelude                                                                  1

2   Introduction                                                             2

3   Premises: Integration Trumps                                             4

4   Clinical Portraits: Between Radiography and Biography                   14

5   Modus Operandi                                                         165

# Chapter 1

# Prelude

### Chronos Is Everywhere

*(Ekphrastic poem about the cover painting by Johan Clarysse)*

A still from a film to show that only man
Knows the duress of time. Whether on
The platform of a subway, the destination
Unknown or at a compulsory reception,
Remotely listening to somebody's
Never-ending speech: a crowd whose
Faces don't matter.

Never mind
The landscape of ghosts, of escape
Gates and scapegoats that remain
Cheaply out of sight.

**Mark Kinet**

DOI: 10.4324/9781003490609-1

# Chapter 2

# Introduction

This book is the English translation, update, and adaptation of the 26th book in the Dutch-language series *Psychoanalytisch Actueel* (Current Psychoanalytics), first published in 2018. This series is intended to be broad and multicultural. It aims to show the theoretical and clinical scope of the psychoanalytic approach within mental health care. It has now established a strong position in the Dutch-speaking landscape. Various topics are reviewed per their profile, each examined in different settings and from different angles. The aim is to show psychoanalysis in its contemporary form.

Unlike the Dutch-language *Tijdschrift voor Psychoanalyse* (Journal of Psychoanalysis), the books are not only read by purely psychoanalytically oriented parties. The books reportedly provide them with helpful inspiration for various forms of mental help. However, people sometimes stumble over technical language or many references that complicate rather than aid the reading. This criticism is understandable. After all, in a way, psychoanalysis may fit a novel text rather than a course text.

In any case, it was an excellent opportunity for an even more clinical book than my previous one, in which jargon is avoided as much as possible and metapsychological or other abstraction is severely limited. In clinical practice, the leading guideline is to *throw away the book*. The patients should open *their* books, and we intend to read and interpret what comes live on stage in the therapeutic space and what is written on and between the lines. In the process, the therapist suspends their knowledge and cleverly keeps a low profile.

My theoretical inspiration and references can be drawn from the first book in my 'trilogy': *Psychoanalytic Principles in Psychiatric Practice. A Remedy by Truth*. The reader can glean from it how I tried to master various psychoanalytic concepts and approaches. It dealt comprehensively with the principles of my practice. It is characterised by integration among the often so divergent psychoanalytic currents that I explained there. The more than 80 pages of notes and references that testified to it will be absent from this book, as I let the clinical situation speak foremost here.

I have now completed more than 30 years of full-time work as a psychoanalytically trained psychiatrist, mainly within a clinical psychotherapeutic

DOI: 10.4324/9781003490609-2

milieu for anxiety, mood, post-traumatic, and personality problems that I have set up and organised myself. I also draw on many years of experience in group psychotherapy, individual psychotherapy face to face, and, to a lesser extent, play therapy and psychoanalysis on the couch. In the first chapter of this book, I summarise the principles of my practice in a few premises.

Barring a few exceptions following written informed consent (see Modus Operandi at the back), I present psychotherapeutic practice in clinical portraits. I call it psychotherapeutic because it illustrates the psychoanalytic scope within a psychiatric practice. I speak of portraits because they are not classical vignettes where psychoanalytic details are zoomed in on but concrete examples illustrating all sides of practice (both in breadth and depth). Finally, in the third part of my trilogy, I will let patients testify about their psychodynamic psychotherapy process in their own words.

Psychoanalytic therapy is still too often—and completely wrongly—identified with the typical cure several times a week on the couch. Persistent feeling, moreover, is that it would only target navel-gazers with luxury problems, whereas it can be fruitfully applied to many forms of (also life-threatening) psychological suffering. All around the world (and, alas, especially nowadays), people can have great trouble surviving warfare, but what about the invisible wars in our families and/or in our inner world?

Writing the portraits presented me with significant challenges. Not only does each patient open their book to a greater or lesser extent, but there is also a whole book to be written about each patient. With each session, new details or facets emerge, shedding a different light on things. Each description is, therefore, only a snapshot—a varying point in time that defines an ever-changing perspective.

There are always multiple ways of looking at the same phenomenon. How can I do justice to clinical complexity while proving or clarifying actual practice? How can I reconcile this with my respect for, and discretion towards, the patient? Of course, I have anonymised as much as possible so that the patients can at most recognise (and hopefully find) themselves in the descriptions or statements.

The portraits are primarily about what was discussed or expressed in the first encounters. To a good listener, they announce (like the overture of an opera) many, if not all, the later themes that will be discussed further. Besides, they are usually the only contacts I note down verbatim.

Under constant bombardment from critics of all kinds, I try to let these portraits speak for themselves. They illustrate the naturalism of the clinical situation, where realism takes precedence over utopianism. Put playfully, the portraits move between radiography and biography. They try to make what is invisible visible, sketching both the life history and its main characters. Together with an ever-unique biological constitution, they decide what the patient makes of their life. As a species, we may all want the same things, but how we try to make this happen, with varying degrees of success (also in symbolic-imaginary ways), is entirely different for each of us.

Indeed, I explicitly thank patients and staff for their trust, not least because we learned a lot from each other's 'mistakes'.

# Chapter 3

# Premises

## Integration Trumps

### Integration

If I had to select the central premise of my practice, I would choose a commitment to integration. Integration involves the thoughtful and coherent connection of initially disjointed or even contradictory contents. In this case, this is done not least by looking for a common stem or root from which they sprout.

Integration is explicitly distinct from a (more superficial) eclectic approach, where different elements are bundled into a whole, lumped together, or juxtaposed without an organising principle. My organising principle is history, as will become clear later. What history underlies what takes place? How have we written and rewritten it? How does it leave its mark on our (inter)actions?

The integration mentioned above materialises in several ways. First: integration of intrapsychic components or forces that are more or less in tension. Classically, in psychoanalysis, there is first the conscious and preconscious, which are separated from the unconscious by an ineradicable (but varying in terms of permeability) repression barrier. Nowadays, from a neuropsychoanalytic perspective, this unconscious is considered essentially a memory system. Structurally or systemically, you have the division between Id, Ego, and SuperEgo. In addition to the inter-systemic, where the Ego has to mediate between the Id, SuperEgo, and the outside world, there are also a lot of intra-systemic conflicts with which the Ego feels itself confronted.

Within the Id, for example, a battle rages between the Ego- or self-preservative drives and the sexual drive or between life and death drives. An essential principle from my *The Spirit of the Drive in Neuropsychoanalysis* is that mutual tensions between seven instinctual systems should be added to this (following Jaak Panksepp and Mark Solms). They form specific neurophysiological and anatomical circuits manifesting in a particular behavioural repertoire we share with mammals. They are, therefore, capitalised: SEEKING/WANTING, LIKING, CARE, ATTACHMENT/GRIEF, LUST, RAGE, FEAR/AVOIDANCE, and PLAY.

Contradictions can also occur within the SuperEgo, where a 'natural' conscience clashes with (sometimes mutually incompatible) commandments,

DOI: 10.4324/9781003490609-3

prohibitions, norms, and ideals. Even within the Ego, it is not all peace. It can, for instance, struggle with different and sometimes conflicting attachments and loyalties; as a result of identification processes, it also contains, for example, the (object-relational) precipitation of our relationships with significant others and their mutual conflicts.

Second, integration refers to gathering and intertwining different theories or concepts from psychoanalytic thought. The first book of my trilogy deals with them all in more detail: drive theory and Ego psychology, object relations theory and self-psychology, and attachment theory in connection with mental processes and their respective neuropsychoanalytic correlates. Depending on the patient and the moment, the psychoanalytic spectrum employed ranges between Anglo-Saxon relational psychoanalysis and more or less linguistically tinged Lacanian counterpoints.

Third, it is about integrating through the judicious use of various lateral disciplines or giving other visions of psychology and psychopathology their complementary or supplementary place and value within an (essentially tragic) psychoanalytic view of man. Biological and psychological treatment, pharmacotherapy, and psychotherapy are not mutually exclusive. They play a leading or secondary role depending on the patient or the moment. Pharmacological treatment of major mood disorders can be combined with a psychoanalytic approach. Conversely, pharmacotherapy can modulate unbearable moods, thus making psychotherapy possible. My earlier book discussed and argued the difference between psychiatric and psychodynamic pharmacotherapy.

Within the psychotherapeutic approach, an insight-*taking* attitude does not prevent other, different from insight-*giving* techniques either. If symptoms (e. g. eating disorders, phobias, or obsessive-compulsive behaviours) are too life-threatening or debilitating, action should be taken not only on experience but also on or through behaviour. Problems often arise in a systemic context. This environmental context can contribute to their origin and persistence, and this context should, therefore, be included in treatment. After all, psychoanalysis has no monopoly over the human mind or the unconscious. At times, its '*follysophy*' can even have a common ground with philosophy. Cognitive science and neuroscience, empirical observational or experimental research, ethology and primatology, and developments such as artificial intelligence can all shed added light on its cause.

In its more social sense, integration involves accommodating or including oppressed or isolated minorities in the broader population. In this form of integration, encounter and dialogue prove to be the most effective remedy against stranger anxiety and the more or less drastic expulsion or scapegoating phenomena that can accompany it. Also, living under our skulls, to some extent, are all sorts of figures or representations that can be pushed away or split off. The return of what was pushed away or split off sooner or later leads to symptoms or acting out behaviour. Now and then, as if out of nowhere, a little devil appears out of a box, or a corpse falls out of the closet.

In these domestic affairs, striving for integration is also the order of the day—striving because it ultimately involves a kind of mission impossible. Humans are and stay divided. They are sick animals. They are essentially disharmonious, marked by language. From a psychoanalytic point of view, perhaps the most characteristic aspect of drive, trauma, and their fates is that they can never be (fully) integrated.

## Clinical Psychotherapy

I am a psychiatrist, and clinical psychotherapy has been my main field of activity for over 30 years. In terms of therapeutic policy, I try to promote an integration between psychiatry, psychotherapy, and psychoanalysis. Within indirect patient care, this involves various forms of teamwork. Within direct patient care, there is weekly 'psychoanalytic process counselling', individually and in groups, weekly living group and ward meetings, and a patient–staff meeting. Specifically, simultaneous pharmacotherapy and psychotherapy, group and individual psychotherapy, psychoanalytic therapy, and behavioural or family therapy in clinical psychotherapy, thus conceived, are no exception. The former can create a framework or enabling conditions for a lot of so-called 'psychiatric patients' to achieve a psychoanalytic process.

The term 'psychoanalytic process counselling' refers to a specific type of guidance offered in a clinical setting. The psychotherapeutic work is conducted by psychoanalytically trained psychotherapists, individually and in groups. The psychiatrist in charge monitors and guides the therapeutic process and patients' current actions, individually and in groups. The psychiatrist's role is to provide commentary, explanations, motivation, and therapeutic process facilitation, make necessary adjustments, or set boundaries.

Of course, how to live their life concretely cannot be decided in the patient's place. On the other hand, the psychoanalytic process is an operation in which things only work under specific conditions. When the patient is groping around in the dark on all fours (sometimes wandering and desperate), we are not afraid to help and guide them. After all, thanks to psychoanalysis, we are undoubtedly familiar with the multitude of mental complexes and processes as well as with what a psychoanalytic process entails. Some patients continue in psychotherapy with me after their clinical psychotherapy. The vast majority continue to consult with me for psychiatric and psychoanalytic process counselling and continue psychoanalytic psychotherapy with a psychologist with a (sufficiently) similar therapeutic thrust to mine.

The clinical psychotherapy milieu is an unnatural or artificial environment offered mainly in the order of months to people with anxiety, trauma, mood, and personality problems. Most patients continue psychotherapeutic out-patient treatment for a considerable time afterwards (often for several years). More technically, it is said that, throughout the week, all activities, therapies, and encounters are geared towards psychotherapeutic goals such as growth and development, insight and recovery. In other words, it is psychotherapy *through* and not only *in* the hospital setting.

The environment under discussion is not only social but also special. It resembles our early childhood mother-environment, which revolves entirely around us and our inner world. In an ordinary course of events, this mother-environment responded almost seamlessly to our evolving needs with extra-ordinary emotional attunement. She also immersed us—*basso continuo*—in a loving bath of language. Suppose we have been allowed to live this simulta-neously extraordinary and mundane experience. In that case, we have, so to speak, fallen like Obelix into a barrel full of magic potion that strengthens and protects us for the rest of our lives. The result is a basis of enduring resilience and a genuine and creative self, thanks to a secure attachment and mentalising ability, intertwined and playing a critical protective role.

Clinical psychotherapy is an intensive treatment in which the therapy pro-gramme is offered as *work*. People thus face difficulties or limitations. These are stumbling blocks to self-knowledge and sources of resistance of all types. However, unlike the therapist's resistance, their analysis contributes sub-stantially to awareness.

It is a form of treatment that thoughtfully links various perspectives: psychiatry, with its symptoms as a sign of disease to be combated, psy-chotherapy in the form of various psychic influences, and psychoanalysis, which conceives the symptom in its unique way. For psychoanalysis, it is an involuntary, repetitive phenomenon whose meaning is not understood by the person concerned and even less by the environment and it is an attempt at self-help. For this reason, it provides both some gain and loss. Ultimately, psychoanalysis considers the symptom as a signifier or narrative element. It can only be understood and worked on within the *context* of history and/or the therapeutic relationship.

Those who suffer physically get themselves cared for, but those who suffer psychologically try to hide. Usually, only those who can no longer 'hold on' in daily life and functioning enter (semi)residential treatment.

Inpatient practice—more than outpatient practice—also addresses an unselected patient population that sometimes does not even initially ask for psychotherapy. While, in outpatient psychotherapy, only specific sides of the patient and their problems are expressed, in inpatient psychotherapy, a per-sonality unfolds more in its totality. After all, almost the whole of the patient's life happens under a team's watchful and reflective eyes and ears for a long time.

Patients live and work with team members and fellow patients, individually and in small or large groups. There is talking, dreaming, dancing, playing, drawing and painting, music-making. The patient is invited to create and recreate, work and relax. Together, we scrutinise their experience and actions and try to discern the constants and determinants of their bio-psycho-social life. Psychoanalysis, after all, is the science of the unreasonable.

## Psychoanalytic Psychotherapy

Virtually all patients who undergo (semi)residential inpatient psychotherapy follow an outpatient course afterwards, which for many extends over several years. For most, psychoanalytic therapy takes place with a psychologist, and they come for psychiatric and psychoanalytic process counselling consultations monthly. A minority are in psychoanalytic psychotherapy with me, either in weekly group psychotherapy or individually.

In a one-liner, psychoanalytic psychotherapy involves using your reason to understand your feelings and (over)sensitivities. Like the irrationality of slips, dreams, and all kinds of hassles or symptoms, feelings have their rationale on closer examination. This rationale corresponds, however, more to the associative logic of the unconscious than the generally accepted logic of so-called 'common sense'.

Non-specific or generic factors similar to the early parent–child relationship and specific psychoanalytic work are present in the psychotherapy (clinical or otherwise) described here. Specifically, there is and remains a sustained focus on three classic psychoanalytic issues. First, resistance is the *deep down inside* not wanting/not being able to know or not wanting/not being able to change. Second, the set of past (more or less fantasised) experiences act as invisible glasses through which we view the world. Third, there is, of course, the hypothesis of the dynamic unconscious.

What is meant by this dynamic unconscious is not the descriptive unconscious of processes or activities that elude our awareness and whose importance is recognised today both inside and outside psychoanalysis (e.g. by cognitive science and neuroscience). Nor is it about the preconscious that is relatively effortlessly (i.e. without resistance) retrievable—for example, a name or telephone number that is not readily available. The Freudian (dynamic) unconscious is pre-eminently what insists or imposes itself. Sometimes as drive or trauma that demands to be symbolically-imaginatively 'bound', other times as the more or less distorted return of what was once split off or repressed for the sake of various forms of unpleasure. Referring once more to *The Spirit of the Drive in Neuropsychoanalysis*, it is about failing or dysfunctional automation, which needs returning to raw data to achieve different and better symbolisation (so-called memory reconsolidation).

Unlike many other forms of therapy, psychoanalysis does not look to change or improve chemically, magically, or quickly. Instead, it aims to become better through truth, which—fair lasts the longest—looks to produce more lasting effects. Of course, this is not the supposedly objectively correct, scientific truth of *elementary particles* but the personal subjective truth that led French writer Michel Houellebecq to write a novel with the same title. This truth can only be found in our inner world and life history.

Nor is such truth ever exact. Nevertheless, psychoanalysis has a scientific vocation. For instance, even in terms of symptom relief, it can present results equivalent to other therapy forms. This is even though its method does not suit its practice very well, all the more so because it aims to achieve under-lying or structural change rather than mere symptom relief.

While most science is about large quantities and replicability of research, psychoanalysis is, above all, a science of the private. For it, n = 1. After all, it seeks to trace the laws that are situated, or *only* situated, on behalf of this one person. In its view, their unconscious holds the knowledge of repetition—both the repetition of conflictual themes and the repetition of so-called triggers that provoke engulfing non-symbolised or non-mentalised emotions.

Finally, psychoanalytically distinctive is its finality, which in a way can be summed up in the Greek poet Pindarus's famous statement: '*Become who you are*'. It has something at once tautological and incomprehensible. How could you become anything other than yourself? Pindarus encourages Syracuse's tyrant to ignore the people around him. After all, they tell him what to do for selfish or opportunistic reasons. Pindarus invites one to look at one's char-acter. At deep wells that atrophy because one pays too much attention to the opinions of others. Indeed, patients are led to find or become themselves as much as possible. The motto, then, is to grow from one's traits and inner life.

Compelling freedom in the form of the rule of free association aims to bring the patient to full speech. Tristan Tzara from the Dadaist Cabaret Voltaire: '*La pensée se fait dans la bouche.*' Thought is formed (only) in the mouth. The therapist is not a silent figure shrouded in anonymity in this enterprise. He (or she) is not 'a man without qualities'—referring to Robert Musil's famous novel with the same title—but, as in child or play therapy, he moves naturally on the floor or keeps his liveliness like the group psychotherapist. Meanwhile, he relentlessly tries to keep a reflective mode of thinking so that a joint (ad)venture can emerge and develop within the therapeutic encounter.

## Relationship

A hundred years after Freud, psychoanalysis has named, like no other, the so-called non-specific or generic factors that play a fundamental role in any form of therapy. It developed numerous terms and concepts for what happens in the early parent–child relationship, just as the Inuit are said to have a hundred words for snow. It currently attaches great importance to the relationship. For current psychoanalysis, it is a therapeutic agent *in itself*, namely as a womb for psychic developmental assistance. On the other hand, it creates a meeting space where, under transference, our inner self and our past can come *live on stage*.

Another key word in my practice is this (therapeutic) relationship. Just as the parent–child relationship is the matrix within which optimal development can occur, this is also the case for the therapeutic relationship. Ideally, it provides the patient with an environment where safety, grip, and symbolic and mentalising development aid can be offered. Long-term dependency is paradoxically a necessary condition for striving (always rising and falling and with varying degrees of success) for independence. A solid therapeutic relationship, while essential, is, however, also an insufficient condition for treatment. A functional and broad treatment vision is needed to work on mental contents and mental processes in a thoughtful combination of understanding and setting boundaries.

However, providing patients with a reliable and steadfast framework and an address where they feel listened to and understood benefits many. Moreover, the therapeutic relationship and encounter provide a forum where past feelings, sensitivities, and (inter)actions can come on to the scene. They are, alongside evolving historiography, sources of information about the life of the mind, particularly its roots in our (pre)history.

As we know, this prehistory differs from history in that we do not have written sources. It can only be (re)constructed based on archaeological finds. It is written down somewhere, not in the symbolic language of humans but in the analogous language we share with animals. We could compare it to how the annual rings in a tree trunk testify to changing climates and seasons. Respectively, these languages are spoken in our explicit or biographical memory versus our implicit or procedural memory. The latter expresses itself mainly through repeated (inter)action patterns with ourselves and others outside conscious awareness.

In other words, the unconscious previously mentioned also holds representations and experiences that, in a sense, we were never aware of! Not least, they date from this first phase of life, in which our psyche has already taken on decisive folds. They manifest themselves in the form of a *revival* both outside and inside the therapeutic space. They offer a very different source of information to our narrative, which is always and inevitably subject to falsification and/or embellishment. These result from our ongoing pursuit of pleasure and/or avoidance of unpleasure, even at the moment when we want to take our own life.

## Mentalisation and Interpretation

Promoting mentalisation is the next pillar on which my practice is based. What thoughts, feelings, fantasies, and desires underlie our actions? Can we express our mental contents symbolically, or do we try to 'cut' them away in all possible and impossible ways? Can we understand our emotions to some extent, think about them, and share them with others, or do they 'mutely/stupidly' interfere with our physical and psychological functioning? Can we read other people's moods and interpret their actions in a sufficiently nuanced way?

Indeed, our psychic life moves between two poles: mentalisation and evacuation. In the latter, drives and traumas are not mediated by translation but are discharged, shunned, or put into the outside world using all kinds of material or immaterial means. For instance, we may drink, take drugs, flee, injure ourselves, react to our emotions unthinkingly, go into the wild, and so on.

Mentalisation capacity and basic security are two proportional flip sides of the same coin. They decide our resilience, stress resistance, and, to some extent, our immune system. High or limited mentalising ability is, respectively, a protective factor or risk factor par excellence for the most diverse forms of psychopathology.

As a form of therapy, psychoanalytically oriented therapy is classically characterised by interpretation. In a narrower sense, psychodynamically, it is about clarifying emotions or behaviour by understanding them to be the result of conflicting unconscious drives or forces and or making them psychogenetically understandable by relating them to patterns and sensitivities from our history that assert their lasting influence.

Psychoanalytic therapists are constantly looking to explore the workings of the unconscious through specific traces. I am thinking particularly of products of the unconscious, such as the dream, acting out and enactment, the parapraxis or the symptom—at least in the sense described above. They are especially hunting for the latter.

I like to refer in this context to the famous Latin proverb: *errare humanum est, perseverare diabolicum*. To err is human; to repeat is diabolical. The diabolical is (until proven otherwise) indicative of the demonic elements of the unconscious. *Quod analysandum est*. What must be analysed. It is mainly these latter involuntary phenomena that are symptomatic. They run in minor or major red threads/live wires through life.

The only way to make them harmless is to take them apart and analyse them. The fatal repetition in question is always an alloy of two types. We are more or less tangled up with repeating themes or (over)sensitivities. There is the repetition of triggers to which we react repeatedly with raw and stereotypical emotions and behaviour. Breaking through failing and dysfunctional automation requires repeated passage through the conscious to deconstruct and reconsolidate or automate new interpretations and interactions.

Neither less nor more than repetitions of understanding and editing are within the scope of a psychoanalytic approach. The rest is—paraphrasing Freud—ordinary human miseries. Woody Allen sums them up laconically in his feature film *Annie Hall* as 'the horrible and the terrible'. They are always emotionally more bearable with others than alone, though.

Indeed, several other interventions also contribute to the psychotherapeutic process or pave the way. These are the four Cs of clarification, confrontation, construction, and castration. Clarification is the ordering or listing of initially confused or confusing emotional phenomena. After all, besides insight, an overview is also essential. What announces or presents itself as diffuse and unlocalisable malaise is delineated, like the doctor trying to dissect diseased from healthy tissue. This allows you to see the proverbial trees through the forest, again or for the first time.

Sometimes, the patient is unaware of more or less contradictory aspects of their thoughts, feelings, or behaviour. Careful and discreet confrontation is proper when the patient is invited to dwell more on contradiction and/or explore it more deeply.

It often happens that some construction is made after the very first interviews. This involves detecting the signs of the complaints or problems of the current admission and launching a hypothesis that broadly exposes the roots, synthesises them, and makes sense of the issues.

Depending on the 'material' the patient produces afterwards, whether and to what extent this trial construction/interpretation is successful can be estimated. Both the content of the associations and the improvement in contact/deepening of rapport help answer whether we are indeed moving in the right direction immediately.

Just as parenting—like Ulysses—navigates between two whirlpools (the Scylla of appeasement and the Charybdis of frustration), psychotherapy moves between understanding and limiting or between gratification and frustration. The castration spoken of within psychoanalysis, then, is not a veterinary procedure but refers to a paternal *function* (not necessarily executed by a father figure) that lays down the law and draws boundaries and thus both curbs and protects. It ensures, for instance, that the patient does not lose themself in a finally unregenerate pleasure (in Lacanian terms: *jouissance*).

## Emancipation

Kant's motto for the Enlightenment is *Sapere aude*. Dare to think. In any form of psychoanalytic therapy, that becomes: dare to think *out loud*. Look inward and also at what is your 'thing' and what makes you tick. Free yourself from an obscurity for which (only) you are ultimately responsible. This is a project of emancipation where, over time, you will make yourself more autonomous (Greek: *auto-nomos*) in your law. This journey towards autonomy is a testament to the potential for personal growth and empowerment within each of us.

Therapy is like Ariadne helping Theseus out of the Minoan labyrinth, because an obvious exit from the maze is simply the entrance. After all, a beautiful statement Ludwig Wittgenstein made about philosophy also applies to psychotherapy. *How do you show the fly the way out of the bottle?* For that, you have to mentally retrace your steps far enough away and understand and remember well where and why you went down the 'wrong' road. It is a matter of fathoming your history and becoming aware of what you have made of it and by what and by whom you are determined. In a one-liner, you must first see where you ended up to get out. Specific patterns have installed themselves in our psyche throughout our lives, without us realising it. For want of better ones, we keep repeating them. Even when they don't work. What is repeated needs to be remembered. This way, we can try to get to the root of the pattern. The most complex and lengthy phase of any psychoanalytic process is working through. You know what repeats itself emotionally and/or in (inter)action, and you also know why, but you do not get this mechanism broken down into one, two, three. Time and again, you relapse into the same patterns. But the journey of self-discovery is what makes this process intriguing and engaging.

Finally, in this process, you may even bump into a complicated and opaque core. You can keep fighting it and try to make the best of it—for instance, by following this gut feeling and identifying with it. Paraphrasing John Fitzgerald Kennedy: *ask not what you can do for your symptom, ask what your symptom can do for you.* Each person has their thing, each animal its pleasure. Only thus do we become or stay *alive and kicking.*

Life must be understood backwards, but it must be lived forwards. Backwards because, like rowers, we sit with our backs to our destination. We steer guided, as much as anything, by the road behind us. Forwards to make our dreams come true, while sufficiently considering both laws and practical objections. This is a matter of psychoanalytic realism, to be explicitly distinguished from psychoanalytic idealism or utopianism.

## Realism

As a science but also as a movement, psychoanalysis has long strived to preserve its purity. It was fixated on its identity, as it were, which it anxiously tried to protect against all kinds of attacks, alleged or otherwise. One question often asked in the midst of this was whether this was *genuine* psychoanalytic work. The criterion was whether this psychotherapeutic work was following this or that gospel because its ideas were written down in several scriptures that were more or less holy to many. This logic was used to assess whether and to what extent the patient qualified for which alloy of psychoanalysis's gold, and a treatment was conducted that followed the book as much as possible.

In the actual practice under discussion here, logic is reversed to a significant extent. Emotional and subjective truths are touched on in a way and moment that suits the patient's capabilities. Of course, it is substantially at odds with selling fables (including to oneself). But the truths spoken of are handled like oxygen. We need it but cannot breathe it in its pure form.

In practice, the administration of and exposure to this oxygen should be continuously dosed and titrated in a matched manner. After all, the patient can only absorb it if, when, and to the extent that they can use it. Resistance must first be understood before it can be fought.

Clinical portraits follow in the next chapter. Since a person-centred rather than disorder-centred approach is used, they are not divided into various diagnoses such as neurosis, borderline, perversion, psychosis, narcissistic, post-traumatic, or toxicomania problems. That way, unnecessary and often counterproductive '*disorderism*' is avoided. How do patients make up their story and their history? How do they characterise (their interaction with) its protagonists and identify their impact? Indeed, the portraits aim to illustrate the multiple naturalisms of psychoanalytic psychotherapy in psychiatric practice. Above all, they endeavour to be truthful and are stripped of all trappings. That's why they are not all success stories.

# Chapter 4

# Clinical Portraits

## Between Radiography and Biography

### Anita—an Eternal Smile

This 30-year-old woman was referred after she has already been hospitalised twice in the psychiatric ward of a general hospital (henceforth PWGH) owing to depressive symptoms and suicide attempts. After seven years of living alone, she struggles to find meaning in her life. What 'killed' her was the fact that her friends had abandoned her for Christmas. Though she's been in psychotherapy for several months, she still feels emotionally withdrawn and struggles to express her feelings despite claiming she has a good relationship with her parents.

Her father is an electrician. He is described as a lovely, helpful man, but he can be stubborn and never gives in when conflicts arise. She had a lot of fun with him. They went swimming together a lot, walking, and cycling. He was a real playmate; they were 'exactly like two children playing together'. Her mother is an office worker. She would be overprotective and cling to Anita. She feels her mother often smothers her. Still, her mother helps in Anita's household. They frequently go out shopping together in the city. Anita finds it difficult to express herself to her mother. She tends to bottle up everything. 'I nod yes even when I want to say no.' She has a brother who is two years her senior and quite a bit more articulate than she is, and he fought his way free during puberty.

Anita says she had a 'perfect childhood'. In a structured *adult attachment interview*, this idealising description is typical of the avoidant type of insecure attachment. She reports she had a naturally sunny disposition and had many friends. She spent whole days playing outside, as she did not like studying very much. During adolescence, she developed an eating problem. 'I felt too fat, and gradually, this took on more extreme proportions. I starve myself; I feel ugly. All the fat has to go.' She did not like (to see) herself. Things took on threatening proportions: there was forced vomiting, abuse of appetite suppressants and laxatives, and sometimes she fainted from weakness. She wanted to study fashion, but her mother was not too keen.

Anita's idol is Naomi Campbell. Laughing, she notes that she may be as skinny but will never be as black as Naomi. From the age of 19, she became

DOI: 10.4324/9781003490609-4

isolated. She pretended to be content and put on a mask. For instance, she supposedly went out and told her mother she had a good time. In reality, she stayed in the car in a car park and did not return home until midnight. During a summer holiday, she was assaulted by two men, but she never told anyone and got off the plane a few days later with a broad smile. Still in her adolescence, she discovered that she was more attracted to women. She fell in love several times but always kept this hidden from everyone. Only far from where she lives can/does she go out and experiment with lesbian contacts. Only there does she lead her own (albeit hidden) life.

In the forensic world, a culprit is looked for. In psychotherapy, it is about understanding hidden connections. Usually, significant others in the environment are (also) involved somehow. Many can come to realise that psychological problems have something to do with the parents or upbringing. However, few realise to what extent this is often the case. In Anita's case, several factors play a role in varying combinations. To begin with, there is a false-self problem. She has always tried to be everything to her mother: her ideal sunshine that shows no downside and satisfies her mother completely. Unsurprisingly, even in transference (within the therapeutic encounter), Anita always shows herself to be sweet and good-natured. The other side of the coin is that, by virtue of her true self, abandonment, anger, and depression prevail.

Anita often feels neither seen nor understood. She keeps such perceived undesirable content away from contact with others. She is not allowed (even in a sexual sense) to be 'wrong' (with its connotation of homosexuality). Net, this all translates into difficulty speaking. She acts out negative feelings, often lapsing into petulant and unruly behaviour. It is out of her mother's sight and knowledge that she acts out. The father was present as a friend rather than a symbolic, limiting, or normative authority. He did little to fulfil his role as a lawgiver; he did not counterbalance the mother's desire. Thus, he did not ease the path to individuation and sexualisation. Her wings barely developed in the absence of the necessary airspace.

There is something androgynous about Anita. She seems entrenched in the latency phase. Puberty threatened the anxiously kept idyll with her mother. She is also confused and conflicted because of lesbian infatuations. Following the sexual trauma, she blames herself for her complacency and naivety. She cannot forgive herself for not defending herself. Afterwards, she fled even more into the regression of the pre-sexual. She still wants to be a child and hide behind her mother's skirts. There is pronounced anorectic behaviour and excessive fitness. As a result, she loses her feminine curves, messes up her menstrual cycle, and uses accumulated anger as fuel for continuously expending energy motorically.

We can think of this as a kind of substance dependence. Sport is then the means she uses to evacuate unbearable contents instead of mentalising them. Thus, she is running away from her difficulties (literally). She works out on the treadmill until she almost literally collapses.

Anita has been in inpatient psychotherapy for about a year. She is susceptible to the slightest discontinuity in care and attention because of the environmental mother and then shows negative attention-seeking behaviour. She can show her feelings or act them out in one scene or another but has yet to learn to speak the language of feelings. 'Expressive' therapy, which works mainly with collages, provides this impetus.

Underneath the psychotherapeutic process, there is a constantly changing need to hold on and let go that needs to be responded to in a sufficiently attuned way. Conflicting feelings trump this, requiring the therapist's empathic, painstaking work. In the relationship with the mother, it seems as if distance and closeness were dictated more by the mother's evolving needs than Anita's. There was proximity but little emotional attunement. She is also terrified of falling into the other's 'grip' and being passively at the mercy of his sexual power and arbitrariness. Therefore, sufficient 'healthy' aggression is needed to evade 'otherman's' imperatives. If you don't want to be a victim, you have to be able to fight. It is mainly within the transference that Anita, with ups and downs and varying degrees of success, is trying to show her teeth a bit more.

## Mireille—Safest on the Streets

This frail 30-year-old woman was born in Argentina. Her mother was the fifth wife of her natural father, and the patient was his seventh child. When Mireille was five, the mother fled to Belgium with her children because of intra-family violence, and relatives took them in. Since then, Mireille has visited her father once, when she was an adolescent. She stayed with him and his partner for several weeks, but he watched football throughout that period and did not pay her attention. In Belgium, she was taken in by grandparents and various uncles and aunts for a while.

When Mireille was seven years old, her mother remarried, to a Frenchman, who turned out to abuse alcohol and be violent. He tyrannically controlled and terrorised Mireille and was emotionally (sadistically) abusive and 'messed up'. The mother had a severe alcohol problem. She is called a 'slut' by Mireille. She had been on disability for years but was previously a shop assistant. She was very domineering and authoritarian but primarily selfish. She was sexually transgressive and (partly as a result of constant intoxication) negligent. 'She smelled of alcohol, cigarettes and frying fat.' There was material neglect (too little, unhealthy, or spoiled food; unwashed second-hand clothes), educational neglect (no values, boundaries, or rules; Mireille is self-made), and affective neglect.

Mireille was scared of her stepfather and men, as well as conflicts and arguments from childhood. She also had contact eczema. There was a lot of fundamental insecurity, homelessness, and loneliness. On the other hand, there was parentification: Mireille remained solid and brave, managed the household, kept up with chores constantly, and stayed away from home and on the streets for as long as possible. 'Some children feel safest on the streets.'

From the age of 14, Mireille wanted to escape the parental home but did not feel big/independent enough to do so. Following a threesome in which she had to reenact a porn scene with her mother and stepfather, she ran away at the age of 16 with the help of a teacher. Later, she was hospitalised in a psychiatric hospital for a long time, after which, with the support of developmental interventions, she was put on a sound track, was able to start higher studies, build a steady relationship and family, and so on. However, after the birth of her children, she became anxious and insecure and began to doubt her maternal abilities. Diagnosed with postpartum depression, she was hospitalised to a PWGH after her last two pregnancies. Her childhood began to haunt her mind in the form of flashbacks, re-experiences, and nightmares. Once again, she felt haunted and terrorised by her stepfather. He controlled everything, interfered with her intimate hygiene, and arbitrarily changed all kinds of rules so that Mireille did not know what to do or how to avoid his reprisals. Silently and obediently, therefore, she displayed as much 'desired behaviour' as possible.

Mireille has since been in psychotherapy for many years. Full admission was needed initially for her to experience basic safety and protection. She needed a motherly holding and facilitating environment to gain sufficient ground. She made frequent use of the seclusion room at her request because only there did she feel sufficiently out of reach of her pursuing stepfather.

Her story mainly revolved around him initially, and her mother remained largely off the record. When this post-traumatic distress was largely overcome, she resumed her work as a teacher and continued to attend outpatient services twice a week. Gradually, after that, memories and re-experiences of massive abandonment and neglect by her mother came to the fore. Mireille felt helpless and lost. She needed maternal care and had to be re-hospitalised for inpatient psychotherapy.

Whereas, initially, it was sadistic abuse, more memories related to sexually transgressive behaviour surfaced. She then felt she was the plaything/toy of a perverse and sinister couple. To top it off, a memory of a threesome she was involved in when she was 16 emerged.

For several months, she was full of disgust and humiliation between the pincers of her mother's legs and at the mercy of her raping stepfather. She made many drawings and clay work in expressive therapy depicting such (she said) 'porn scenes'. There was almost complete nutritional refusal during this period, resulting in extreme weight loss and a critical general condition. She drank gallons of water to rinse her mouth and throat and cleanse herself as much as possible of all filth.

On closer inspection, she fled the house permanently owing to this experience. However, the sexual trauma was then buried in excessive alcohol and drug use, anorectic-bulimic behaviour, and promiscuous sexual acting-out where she indulged in nightlife and 'played' with (the feelings of) men. When she met her future husband, she was an independent, free-spirited, bold young woman with great grit. There was a great contrast with the very shrunken girl who almost wants to come and sit on her therapists' laps to bask in their warmth and understanding.

Meanwhile, she has got into a cat-and-mouse game with her husband. A stepfather/perpetrator transference towards him has established itself. Feeling controlled and dominated, she raises her middle finger behind his back. By spending a lot of money on clothes, she makes him pay ('Fuck you!') as she manages to evade her stepfather's abuse of power at the time with all sorts of tricks. It is difficult for the husband to sympathise or empathise with Mireille's subjective world. Moreover, he is increasingly hostile to the treatment. Even though she continuously suffers from post-traumatic relapses, he also sexually imposes his will and whims on her.

Mireille undergoes all this idly while silently thinking more and more about divorce and making concrete plans to this end. She is constantly fighting for her own inner life. She runs half a marathon daily: she combines part-time daycare with her work, her household, and caring for her husband and children, and she is on the road for hours by train, bus, and car to spend enough time in our supportive and understanding mother environment.

Clinically, the common observation is that the most significant practical, organisational, or logistical problems are peanuts compared with unmet emotional needs. People are willing and able to move heaven and earth to find a modicum of understanding and acknowledgement. When her husband finally confronts her with the choice of stopping her treatment (he does not like her evolution towards increased disobedience and rebellion) or getting a divorce, she chooses the latter. She properly arranges the divorce, finds a new place to live, resumes work, and juggles impending demotion and co-parenting.

Possibly, in part, in reaction to and defending against separation and abandonment, things degenerated over the following months, first into a hypomanic episode and later into a full-blooded manic-psychotic episode. The second, incidentally, occurred despite the necessary psychopharmaceuticals, including mood stabilisers, that had meanwhile been started *lege artis*. She initially knew of no family psychiatric antecedents for severe mood disorders, but only then did she begin to wonder whether her mother's collecting frenzy, her periods of nocturnal restlessness, and mainly her sexual disinhibition should not also be attributed to mania. Was the debauched period she experienced as a young adult perhaps also an expression of a hypomanic state? Moreover, she learns from an Argentine half-sister that there were two suicides in her father's family.

Over the years since then, she has been coming to see me weekly. A sustained therapeutic relationship, on good and bad days, provides psychosocial stability. Although various aspects of abandonment, neglect, and abuse continue to be discussed and worked on, the major psychiatric mood disorder has gradually come to the fore. The result is loss, loss, loss. Loss of her family, of her work, of her (cognitive and energetic) ability, of her youthful body. Apart from two three-week admissions, however, she manages on an outpatient basis. Fortunately, divorced but with sufficient co-parenting harmony, she has good bonding/contact with her three now young adult children, with whom she seems to have kept strong emotional and communicative bonds. With no other family or relatives around, her oldest daughter (now at university) is invited twice a year to discuss her mother's actions and her mood. Especially in bipolar disorders, minimal hetero-anamnestic data are, after all, essential because hypomania can arise unnoticed and cause considerable damage.

## Rita—a Tough Woman in Soft Hands

On referral from her outpatient psychiatrist, a woman in her 50s is hospitalised after having been in treatment for about three years, including a year in a day centre for work rehabilitation, but, in her own words, 'without results'. At the age of 16, she was first hospitalised in a psychiatric hospital for a week after attempting suicide with an overdose of medication.

Rita is the eldest of three children, and she was born slightly premature: 'I was an incubator child'. For the first six months of life, she was cared for by her maternal grandmother ('my real mother'). It was a big disappointment for the parents that she was not a boy. A sister died of cancer, and there is only superficial contact with the brother. The father died. He was a teacher, and she described him as 'a real monkey'. With tears in her eyes, she says he gave the children more beatings than food. He was a real torturer who also sexually abused Rita and offered her as a sexual exploit to his friends. Her mother is a cafe boss. 'I never had a mother.' She never protected Rita from the ill-treatment of her father, and Rita also received a lot of beatings from her.

Rita has always kept herself solid and brave, splitting off feelings of abandonment and keeping them away from others. During her adolescence, she was more 'for the women' and a bit macho or bad-boyish herself. She had an excellent relationship with her girlfriends. She was in a relationship with a man 15 years older than her and, after two years of courtship, she was also married for about ten years to a man nine years older than her. She has two sons from this marriage, and they are doing well and have mainly made/found their way in life.

Since the divorce, she has had two long-term relationships with women, ending up in a caring role each time. Her current partner, for instance, is paralysed in the lower limbs and 'a dead mouse'. In all her relationships, there was sexual aversion on her part. Therefore, it suits her well that she has nothing to fear from her current partner.

Rita has always been self-employed in the hospitality industry and built quite a bit there as a tough woman, but, as a result of the alcohol and gambling addiction of her children's father, she went bankrupt. She has enormous debts and is trying to manage the last few years on illness benefits. There is chronic denial and splitting off of dependency needs and lifelong post-traumatic symptoms (nightmares, flashbacks) related to sexual polytrauma.

Rita was hospitalised for several months for inpatient psychotherapy. This allowed some 'coming to terms', and there was a hesitant opening in the form of budding recognition of her painful history and feelings. With the onset of trusting relationships with us as a springboard, she was able to start out-patient psychotherapy that has now been running weekly for several years. For the first time, she finds understanding there. Depressive symptoms are subsiding, and, in her voluntary work, she is gradually developing as the driving force of a shelter for behaviourally disturbed children. She runs a cooking workshop there and is named and experienced as a Mother Teresa by the youngsters. This gives her great satisfaction.

Although often very depressed, she never wanted to take psychopharmaceuticals. As a child, she was drugged with the notorious Rohypnol (the 'date-rape drug'), so that she was defenceless and at the mercy of her abusers. She does not want to feel numb in any way, but, paradoxically, she is almost constantly in a mild dissociative state. Only during interviews does this thaw, and feelings of abandonment and traumatic re-experiences come up at intervals. The latter are never made explicit. They appear in allusions and implicit references. An active translating attitude on the part of the therapist is needed to get her story.

There has chiefly been an evolution in terms of basic safety and trust. Rita feels less abandoned and misunderstood. She can access both her psychotherapist and psychiatric and psychoanalytic process counselling, where her SOS and other messages are handled gently and tactfully.

The famous corrective emotional experience is more beneficial to her than insight or classical psychoanalytic work. It is part of the generic or non-specific therapeutic factors of positive acceptance, empathy, predictability, and sustained engagement in good and bad days. Processes of interiorisation and introjection outweigh narrative or interpretive verbalisation. A therapeutic encounter is internalised, creating a more secure attachment and thus increased coping and stress resilience.

## Joseph—between Pasha and Eunuch

This young man in his late 20s was referred from a PWGH service after he had already had several admissions there because of depressive and psychosomatic symptoms (morning vomiting). He had also previously been hospitalised in a psychiatric hospital 'where they flattened me with medication'. He was in a relationship for two years, but, when they decided to live together, problems and conflicts arose. Joseph's parents interfered in their financial affairs, which created a lot of bad blood between the partner and her parents.

Joseph finds little satisfaction in his work as an educator. He is afraid of, and highly annoyed with, management, by whom he feels constantly controlled and targeted. He also struggles to keep authority in the live-in group with behaviourally demanding youngsters who lack motivation or respect for authority. Joseph does find great pleasure in his hobby (playing music). He wanted to continue his music education but was not allowed by his parents: 'Those artists …'. Eventually, he took the entrance exams for a conservatory, but he felt they didn't want anything of him or were angry with him, so he 'passed up' this option. He still greatly admires other performing artists. He dreams of realising a solo performance one day.

At home, Joseph is the youngest of four and the only son. His mother and sisters mothered him, so he grew up mainly in the realm of women. The mother is described as overprotective and patronising. She monopolises him and emotionally claims him for herself. She cannot tolerate him going his own way and discourages all (but especially phallic) initiatives. Joseph feels he has to answer to her for all sorts of things. Apparently, with him, she had few boundaries: as a child, he accompanied her to the toilet, and, until his adolescent years, they used the bathroom together.

How different it was when Father came home! The latter is described as a gruff, authoritarian man. There was very little communication with him. He was silent, and, when he did say something, Joseph experienced his actions as severe, oppressive, and destructive. He never experienced warmth or affection from his father. His feelings towards him were manifestly hostile. Overall, he felt he could not be himself with his parents. They are reproachful and regard him as ungrateful and spoilt.

As a child, he was said to have been 'hyperkinetic'. Mother gave him a syrup for this. He felt very restricted in his movements. It was exactly like a 'mole hole'. He would have been an overactive and impulsive rascal who knew no danger and was a busy bee. From puberty onwards, he became a lot less so. Around that age, he reportedly developed BDSM fantasies. He dressed up as a schoolgirl, looked at himself in the mirror, fantasised about the girl being punished, and slapped himself on the buttocks in the process. He used his mother's and sisters' lingerie for this role play and feared being caught.

Partly as a result of these 'weird' and clandestine sexual activities, he doubts his masculinity. He is afraid of being considered female or homosexual, complains of insufficient male physicality (e.g. beard growth and body hair), and so on. He also finds himself insufficiently enterprising and actively conquering. For instance, he was told by a music teacher that he would 'not have enough balls', which has stuck with him a lot.

Joseph was hospitalised three times over several months for inpatient psychotherapy. He repeatedly experienced a borderline-psychotic state characterised by anxiety, confusion, diminished consciousness, sexual disinhibition, and sensitive delusion in which he felt rejected or condemned by others. In each case, this state cleared up quickly with low-dose antipsychotics. Content could be discussed and analysed afterwards as in a waking dream. This corresponds to the (now obsolete) diagnosis of hysterical psychosis.

Since these admissions, he has been in outpatient psychotherapy for about 15 years, first weekly and, in recent years, monthly. A metaphor that often came up was that of himself as a eunuch in the harem. When the father/sultan was absent, he delighted in female love and attention. There is also a feminine identification cherishing 'soft' and passive values. There was a sexual over-stimulation that made him sensitive to female beauty/nudity early on. This led to guilt-laden masturbation fantasies in which he simultaneously spanked the girl he stage-managed as himself.

Sometimes, he indulges in exclusive female attention for his phallic exploits and exhibitionism; other times, he hides his 'tail' between his legs with much pent-up anger and hatred towards the all-powerful father. At work, he is afflicted both by the wanton behaviour of pupils and the exercise of power by manage-ment. While he harbours fantasies of murder or manslaughter (his father), he has the most significant difficulty asserting himself or standing his ground.

Over the years, a whole series of women pass by. Either they are women who willingly go along with his craving for sexual games (joint visits to erotic shops, use of sex toys, BDSM fantasies) and who slavishly obey the commandment: 'Blowjob!' Often, these partners are a bit too free and independent for him; they also interact with other men, and he starts to feel insecure and separation-anxious compared with these rivals. Or they are women who offer him security and maternal concern but are less libertine or kinky in the bedroom.

It is never a case of 'everything to his liking'. So, he keeps looking for the all-good mother who gives and grants him everything. In recent years, he has hardly had any problems at work. He has a stable relationship and succeeds better than ever in assuming a paternal role and position vis-à-vis a stepchild he had previously long considered an annoying rival to Mother, the wife.

## Julie—Mad Meg (de Dulle Griet)

This 30-year-old mental health worker is hospitalised because of problems that she says have been dragging on for a long time. She has been in out-patient psychotherapy for some time, but apparently without satisfactory results for her. She lives with her parents again after having had several rela-tionship adventures. Each time, she is left with a 'kind of resentful hangover'.

Recently, she has been shown the door by her father. Consequently, she is distraught and in a bad mood. She has negative feelings towards both par-ents, but especially towards him. On the other hand, her story shows that he took care of her in the early years of her life. Still, he would have preferred a son, and so she fell out of favour when her younger brother was born. The father thinks Julie should have quietly married and found her way. She describes him as a complicated man who is intolerant. He is a 'nag' and a 'negativist'. As a result of his profession, he was absent a lot because he was away from home working. He also has a substantial alcohol problem. In addition: 'I think he has problems with women'.

Mother suffers from anxiety and depression; she does not know what she wants. She suffers from 'learned helplessness', according to Julie. She feels that her mother has used her as an emotional crutch. 'Mum needs me to get her heart out'. Mum lost her mother when she was eight years old and thus missed a mother herself. There is a brother four years younger with whom she was very close until puberty. They sought support from each other because neither of them felt understood by their parents. On the other hand, the latter both act a bit like victims. Julie often feels inadequate, resentful, hurt, and aggrieved, maybe especially as a woman. She then behaves like a Mad Meg/Dulle Griet, usually going to war against all kinds of injustices (perceived or not).

For over a decade, Julie has been in psychotherapeutic treatment. She started with a year of inpatient psychotherapy. Her catty and combative attitude made her constantly the centre of conflicts in the treatment group. She tried to monopolise the group's attention in many ways and reacted jealously when (predominantly female) fellow patients snatched attention away. Towards the men, she was seductive to the point of provocation. She responded furiously and with resentment to the slightest frustration and would then go around wildly and kick up a lot of trouble.

On the one hand, there was a basis of feelings of abandonment. She often felt misunderstood or mistreated. Over time, she became aware of a confident narcissistic posturing in this. After all, unconsciously, she claimed to be treated royally by everyone. There was a combination of great sibling and Oedipal rivalry. The theme of men being slightly superior to women was also a thorny issue.

All this resonated with her history: how she had felt like her father's darling; how she had felt ousted from the throne by her brother and rejected by her father (this repeated itself following an argument in which she was thrown out of the door); how the family consisted of four children and thus resembled a nest filled with four birds with beaks wide-open because they were starving, and how each one remained 'hungry' to a greater or lesser extent.

During admission, she forged a passionate relationship with a fellow group member. By grasping the connection with her history, the storm of negative feelings subsided, and she was able to return to work and outpatient therapy. The end of her residential treatment was entirely dominated by a 'forbidden' passionate love affair with a fellow group member with whom she experienced days of wine and roses. They disregarded ward rules and petty laws, which they lustily flouted as a splendid couple.

Afterwards, she entered weekly outpatient group psychotherapy for several years. The relationship described above lost its lustre as soon as they left our arena. Since then, she has had a few more relationships. She would enjoy being treated by her partners to various exclusive holiday destinations but at once lapsed into discontent if this treatment was not maintained.

For a long time, she identified with the young people/patients rather than the parent figures/helpers in her professional environment. Towards the latter, she stayed pretty hostile. This is probably why they regularly ignored her in extra-professional initiatives, further fuelling her negative feelings.

She has been in a stable relationship with a very old divorced husband and father for the past few years. She needed a lot of time before she could fully commit. After all, she remained on the lookout for another, better partner. Meanwhile, she has chosen him, but it frustrates her that he does not exercise enough authority over his young adult children, who still live with him. Does Julie come first for him? Are her rights wronged? Aren't her stepchildren taking up too much space in their father's heart and home? She can talk about it with humour and perspective. Meanwhile, she is well aware of a similar daily struggle that once took place within her family of origin.

## Hilda—Mega Mindy

This woman, in her late 20s, was referred from a PWGH service because of long-standing anxiety and panic attacks. 'I dare not be alone.' For about two years, she has also had compulsive thoughts: 'I would hurt people. Especially people I love'. During the introductory interview, she lets slip that she 'expresses tremendously positive feelings'. She always keeps herself spirited and robust. She wants everything to go well everywhere. Negative feelings—as it turns out—are never, ever expressed.

Hilda has a senior administrative management position. Her job frustrates her: she has many tasks and responsibilities but cannot make decisions. She feels hurt and short-changed by her director. She has already had a stretch of psychotherapy with a female psychotherapist, but she is angry because she allegedly received insufficient attention and comfort from her.

Hilda is the eldest of three children. She has 'a tremendously good relationship' with the parents. Father is a blue-collar worker. 'I love him greatly.' As a little girl, she was carried in his hands. He also loved to go out with her, showing her off to friends and colleagues. 'He went out with me more than with mum.' She also recounts, for instance, how fine the two of them were when Mum was in the maternity home for the birth of her younger brother. Hilda always thought it was her fault if the parents had arguments or tensions. She was also sometimes explicitly told by her mother to go and appease her father and thus mediate their mutual conflicts.

Mother is initially described as a somewhat bossy woman. But, when Hilda was difficult or naughty, her mother did not get angry but sad. She cried. Hilda felt very guilty. She was also told a lot that her mother had gained a lot of weight as a result of her pregnancy, and that her belly had become a 'battlefield' of stretch marks because of her.

By her admission, Hilda was a cheerful and vibrant child. She endeavoured to be an angel. During her adolescence, Hilda hardly rebelled. However, she did have some unpleasant sexually transgressive experiences that would leave some mark on her further psychosexual development. Thus, she is always careful about potentially 'provocative' clothing and, to this day, never touches a drop of alcohol for fear of losing control and then behaving 'sluttily'.

After six years of courtship, she married a partner who was like an ideal son-in-law to her mother. With him, she mainly sought security and stability.

She was never really in love with him. She could not return to her parental home fast enough the day after her marriage. Until her wedding day, she had slept in the same bed with her mother. Hilda had little appetite for sex, and, when it happened, she had little use for it. She did have an 'affair' a few times. Then, she did get excited and could enjoy sex. Afterwards, however, it left her with a big hangover.

During the clinical psychotherapeutic admission period, she became aware that she could no longer bear to be her mother's angel. She got in touch with anger and other negative feelings that she had always anxiously and compulsively hidden from her mother. In the ward, she rebelled and, feeling like she was at boarding school, indulged in all kinds of vices. She was initially strongly inhibited and/or withdrawn, but her temperament reared its head, and she turned out to be a dazzling woman who dared to be bold in all kinds of small and large group meetings, for instance. Eventually, she even fell in love with a much younger, tough, *bad boy* with whom she started a forbidden relationship (forbidden by both the department rules and her mother).

Hilda underwent an period of clinical psychotherapy lasting about a year and a half. She left in good spirits and went back to work at once (and has worked continuously since). For the first few years, she came in for weekly psychoanalytic group psychotherapy. Since then, for about a decade, she has been coming individually. Often, this is monthly, but, at times, the frequency of sessions is pushed up to weekly or twice a week when she encounters something and wants to explore it further. With her, the psychoanalytic process proceeds in serial or episodic form. It is a format that does occur more often in practice, as a psychoanalytic process sustained from A to Z is more the exception than the rule with many (former) 'psychiatric patients'.

It has been made abundantly clear over time that she experiences many angry and even murderous impulses that she covers under a thick cloak of love. The return of what was repressed leads to obsessive symptoms such as aggressive or sadistic compulsions towards 'innocent people'. She has a particularly hard time with delicate, squeamish figures, . She acts overly empathic and caring towards them precisely because they (like her mother) get on her nerves. 'I would sometimes stick them against the wall.' On the other hand, in professional life or traffic, for instance, she is a very combative and challenging woman who sometimes looks for trouble to vent accumulated aggression, but against total strangers.

Initially, she instead saw herself as a victim of her mother's emotional blackmail. She felt defenceless against her tears, which she saw as a powerful and effective weapon. Based on her stories, the mother appears to be a self-centred woman with low self-esteem. From an early age, Hilda felt 'called' to cheer her up and be her sunshine. She had a vital role in her mother's self-esteem and had to constantly affirm her as a fantastic mother. After school, hot chocolate would await her until puberty, which she was supposed to drink with her mother, whereas she gradually came to prefer to hang out with friends and girlfriends (with or without mopeds) at the school gate. While she is or *should be* there for her mother, in moments of emotional distress, she feels misunderstood and/or abandoned by her mother, as if it is always just *her mother's* feelings that are most important.

In addition to these pre-Oedipal components, Hilda became more aware of rival feelings towards her mother over the years. Secretly, she triumphed over her mother and enjoyed being able to wrap her father (as well as other father figures) around her finger. There are unconscious feelings of guilt and a need for punishment for the harm she caused her mother. She is gradually coming to terms with the fact that she was immensely seductive but in a subtle, hidden way. She often referred to wearing white male vests in which she looked boyish but which showed off her assets to the male crowd just fine.

In therapy, she is susceptible to empathic deficits. This can be linked to how she always experienced her mother. Because of repeated assaults, she was able to detach herself from her *bad boy* shortly after her admission. Her current partner aided her with this. There was/is a 'smell' about him, too (he is a cannabis-smoking, unemployed person who is bogged down in idleness at home, but functions positively as a husband by the fire, offering security). On the other hand, he depends on her and 'carries me in his hands' (an expression she also used for her father).

To him, Hilda is above all women and, therefore, has no competition. Both Oedipal prohibition, punishment, the need for emotional care, and narcissistic gratification find their apparent satisfaction in this symptomatic choice of partner for a time. For Hilda, these cards were on the table, but, for years, it was her 'conscious' choice, so to speak, to play this game with them.

Meanwhile, her partner's cannabis addiction was steadily escalating. For once, he embodied the fragile and squeamish mother who had to be cared for like some puppy in distress (she, nota bene, often brought puppies into the house). We could gradually figure out that these puppies involved an otherlike or alter ego. Then he stood for the father by whom she felt loved, cherished, and adored and who waited with her in the evening with candles and tea lights.

Hilda showed indestructible cheerfulness in our conversations. She stayed away for extended periods. Afterwards, it was always clear that there had been incidents of aggression involving her partner, with him threatening murder and suicide, and she sometimes had to take refuge with the neighbours. It was as if (as towards her mother) she only wanted to show herself at her best to me and solve all her problems alone.

As she spoke, it gradually became clear how terrorised she was. She went to work full-time, ran all the errands, and managed all practical matters because of her partner's social anxieties. She had chronic money problems because he let so much money go up in smoke (literally), and she sometimes had to put herself at risk looking for his 'stuff' in not-always-safe environments.

Meanwhile, she kept hidden from the outside world (not least her parents) how big the problems were. She compared herself to a fairy who could do magic, or Mega Mindy, a kind of wonder woman who plagued youth channels then. Most of all, she was afraid of being accused of it all being her fault. Why did she let it get this far? Why didn't she move away from her partner when she would have been better off staying with her husband instead of leaving him for 'wrong' men?

After yet another threat, which required the intervention of a coincidentally visiting colleague and the police, her partner was finally hospitalised. He went through long-term rehab treatment and had since been working for the first time since being with Hilda. He is still clean and exemplary in his attitude towards and treatment of Hilda. He seems to realise (and also want to make up for) what he has done to her all this time.

While Hilda remained symptom-free all this time, in recent months, she suffered a relapse. First of all, many people only suffer after the war. As long as it is going on, they are in a fight/flight or survival mode, and there is neither time nor space to dwell on their inner selves. The external enemy and hostilities demand all their attention and energy. Hilda develops all kinds of physical complaints, only in 'peacetime' (and thus in delayed reaction), that are considered post-traumatic stress symptoms by her GP.

Another element is that she gets 'tangled up' with her anger again. Just when there is little to criticise about her partner's behaviour, she may become furious in response to all sorts of 'triggers' that remind her of the past terror and nightmare. One 'wrong' word or reaction then suffices for her to feel intense anger and hatred rising within her. She suppresses these feelings because, in her judgement, they do not fit the current state of affairs. However, this 'avenges' in the form of a resurgence of aggressive and troubling compulsive thoughts. They scare her so much that she sometimes fears going mad and having to be hospitalised in a psychiatric hospital again after all these years of 'functioning well'.

Meanwhile, because of their reduced mobility, her parents moved into a flat, and her father died a short time later. Hilda described her mother, in the period of illness leading up to his death, in similar terms as before: self-centred and uninvolved. She did a whole story about a garden gnome she had once gone to buy with her father. To her, he embodied both their poetic-romantic attitudes and the special rapport that existed between father and daughter. Mother had never understood very much about such things. Because she had, without much ado, removed the garden gnome from the balcony of their terrace and put it in the 'big trash', she was portrayed as a heartless but also superficial creature who wholly ignored the finer expressions of the life of the mind.

It is remarkable how her view of her parents has changed since then. Indeed, her mother has appeared as a *lusty widow* in recent years. Despite her advanced age, she is more coquettish and feminine than ever. She also goes 'out' often, visiting museums, the theatre, and even exotic cities and regions.

Hilda has had many conversations with her mother and, as a result, has had to adjust her image of her parents drastically. Her parents dated for a long time and had a very passionate relationship. They waited a long time before having children because they wanted to enjoy each other for longer. The mother had to stay home, under pressure from the father, to take care of the children. The father worked away a lot and left all the child-rearing labour to his wife. He only did enjoyable things with and for the children. He suffered if he wasn't given exclusive attention and could sulk and be stubborn in childish ways. Hilda then felt called (and, in time, she was also required by her mother) to mediate, break the ice, and help her father over the bridge.

More and more, Hilda concluded that she felt guilty just for *being* there. That her birth had made her parents unhappy, and that her mission was to make up for this unconscious 'crime'. She did this by wanting to be her father's princess and mother's angel. On closer inspection, she had been engaged in something of a *mission impossible* all her life. The price she paid for it was that all negative/inappropriate feelings had to be kept hidden and only expressed in compulsive thoughts with a high *Fuck!* content.

She begins one of the sessions by saying:

> I should be happy. My husband goes to work; he doesn't use drugs any-more, and he is sweet and considerate. But I am bored. I think it's a bit boring. He has had a strict routine for the past few months. Have a cup of coffee after work, smoke a few cigarettes, watch some cycling, cook ela-borately, prepare his packed lunch for the day after, then watch some tele-vision together, have a little sex and go to sleep by ten o'clock at the latest.

I am reminded of Arthur Schopenhauer's famous statement that life oscillates like a pendulum from suffering to boredom. Either you desire, and there is a lack, or you seem to have everything you want. You have an appointment with happiness, but happiness doesn't show up. This is an excellent example of the difference between philosophical and psychoanalytical thought. The former is universally human, while the latter looks to uncover the more pro-found and always singular foundation of things.

This is why I allude to the well-known Flemish TV journalist Rudi Vranckx. When he briefly returns to Belgium, he is already longing for some war zone, to which Hilda says, 'Might I be addicted to tension?' I was indeed thinking about her playing with boundaries on the edge of prohibition, which had also been demonstrated many times by a flirtation and (unfinished) mating dance with a married colleague at work that had been going on for years.

Then she tells me she wants to go swimming with the dogs. Her partner said: 'No, sweetie, I don't feel like it'. She is internally furious about this. All these years, she has been super flexible and has at once responded to his sometimes very capricious requests and needs, and now *she* is asking for something! I could react to her story in many ways but prefer to point out a constant. After all, isn't it the problem that she continually adapts entirely to other people and wants to please them? Does she automatically sacrifice her pleasure for that of the other person and does not want to hurt or disappoint them? Several associations follow, illustrating this pattern. To conclude, imagine if you had just said 'No, sweetie' to your mother's request to have a hot chocolate together! With some hilarity, the point seems made with that.

In one of the following sessions, she complains about her relapse in symptoms. Two things upset her. She read in the newspaper about the Romanian killer of a young woman found on the beach in Knokke. He had requested a polygraph test in an attempt to prove his innocence. However, he had failed this test, and further compelling, incriminating evidence was found. Hilda wondered: is it possible to commit a crime of which you are entirely unaware? This thought kept her preoccupied and very scared all weekend.

Her eye had also fallen on a newspaper article that said that research had shown that psychopaths like R&B and hip-hop. Two popular songs from these genres were mentioned and were Hilda's favourites! The thought of being a bit of a psychopath herself did not leave her for days. Reasonable arguments could not dispel this thought. Compulsive thoughts, like all symptoms, are involuntary and cannot be corrected by any reasoning.

The following session was about how, at his request, she orally satisfied her partner, a task she has been painstakingly performing, even over all those years when she experienced hell with him. As she was sucking him ('I kissed him in that place'), she thought of her father's tiny penis. Bedridden and frail, he had lost some propriety at the end of his life, and she had to touch and hide this little penis. Hilda feels anxious and guilty about this association, while her partner and a friend have since put this into perspective to ease her conscience. As a girl, shouldn't she also have made her father's small penis swell? After all, why did he need to appear in public with her? Even then, did she not go out of her way to please him as much as possible?

We are now several years on, and Hilda is currently in psychotherapy twice a week. Why has she tried to turn into a Mega Mindy? Since childhood, she has felt guilty, which makes her want to make up for/repair damage (to her mother and her parents' relationship). At the same time, she stays stuck in a sometimes tricky/painful/degrading relationship with a man her mother disapproves of. Impulses of negative feelings are repelled and underlie sporadic and frightening compulsive thoughts. She fears that inside her is a psychopath, so to speak, who cruelly preys on innocent children.

Classically Freudian, the Oedipus complex plays a crucial role in neurosis. This complex is then taken to mean the set of amorous desires and hostile feelings the child experiences towards their parents. These desires and feelings persist in the unconscious (towards others experienced as parental figures). They can then lead to all kinds of intrusive feelings of rivalry, jealousy, competition, and/or sexual desires for 'forbidden' or 'impossible' partners. They also trigger all sorts of psychological problems, with sexual and narcissistic pleasure being hampered by inhibitions, symptoms, and fears of all kinds. Feeling important, valued, or loved, or feeling good about oneself as a man or woman and enjoying all sorts of things are then disrupted or hindered by unconscious feelings of guilt/punishment.

Although the Oedipus complex rarely appears in contemporary publications, its 'appearance' often forms the final piece of the psychoanalytic process. Only when the whole picture comes into sharp focus is the picture of the problem fully developed, and everything comes together in a broader context and greater relief. A psychoanalytic cure several times a week is an exception today. Many times, the psychoanalytic process takes place at a much lower frequency. As a result, both the manifestations of the Oedipus complex and infantile sexuality come under the magnifying glass much later. The actuality of her incipiently demented mother, the perils surrounding her partner who is using cannabis again (and whom she is trying to divorce for a second time), and incredibly stubborn defences still lead to an arduous analysis of the roots of her obsessive and relational symptomatology despite the current frequency.

### Sara—away from under the Knife

This woman has been in the doldrums for many years with difficult-to-objectify pain symptoms for which multiple surgical procedures (including hip replacement), as well as treatment in various pain clinics, have already been performed. She already had several admissions to various psychiatric settings, all without much result. She begins the interview by saying she was raped three times eight years ago and has never been able to talk about or process this. Apart from her husband and herself, only her parents are aware but take it very lightly: 'What's done is done'.

The case appears to involve an immediate superior in whom she had initially placed great trust and with whom she enjoyed a playful and familiar relationship for a while. He repeatedly lured her into an unprotected and isolated position, after which he violently raped her. Afterwards, he unabashedly and triumphantly expressed himself using derogatory terms about her. So many years after the 'facts', he continues to pursue her and intimidate her with his brutal presence.

Sara works in the healthcare sector and, after five years of courtship, is married to a slightly older man who holds an executive position in industry. He travels and is out of the country a lot with work. She describes him as a tall and robust figure. Because of his mother's suicide during a psychiatric hospitalisation, he is very sceptical about and hostile towards psychiatric treatment. They have four still-school-aged children who manifest no problems.

Sara, the younger of two, has an older brother who is fine in all areas of his life. Father is described as someone powerful. He, too, has a managerial position in the corporate world. He is an athletic go-getter who wants to lead everything, impose his opinion on others, and interfere with anything and everything. We were also able to experience his interference during treatment. He is outspokenly against psychotherapeutic treatment, which he also finds ridiculous.

The mother was said to be a calmer, more docile type who works in the care sector. Sara has always been very controlled by their father, is very docile and compliant, and has never dared to oppose him in any way. From an early age, she was insecure and not resilient at school. 'I let everyone dominate me, and I was an easy target.'

Sara has since been in psychotherapy for several years. Initially, she kept somatising. She went medical shopping and walked in the door of various orthopaedists and anaesthetists. Time and again, examinations were done, as well as significant pain and other treatments. However, objective findings were limited and did not bring much relief. All this while she has vaginal lesions from her rapes, which make her feel 'mutilated'. She dares not show these to anyone, has been to the door of a gynaecologist several times, but always flees.

In addition, she heavily self-medicated, often walking around dizzy because she was under the influence of sedatives. From the outset, it was clear that her pain symptoms (in the hip and pelvic region) were mainly post-traumatic. Admittedly, she had complaints beforehand, but, as in conversion, the pain was attached primarily to this pre-existing somatic problem.

The parents, and especially the father, attached little importance or belief to the rapes and mostly denied any connection to her problems. They constantly resisted psychiatric and psychotherapeutic treatment and insisted on referral for further physical therapy. Several times, the father contacted us on the phone and, on several occasions, he tried to force a meeting unexpectedly and without an appointment. When a scheduled meeting went ahead, he thoroughly lectured us as practitioners.

Meanwhile, his daughter complained to everyone who wanted to hear about our lack of care and understanding. Abandonment feelings were trumped up, and all arrows were pointed at the team. It took a long time before she addressed her rapes. She looked up to how an older colleague had guided her. He continued to take pleasure in chasing her down her street.

Gradually, Sara came out of the corner and tried to signal to employers and human resources departments the perpetrator's sexually transgressive behaviour (even repeated towards other female colleagues). The more she spoke about her revenge, the more she showed various disturbances of consciousness (confusion, blackouts, complete loss of consciousness). If repeated, this would land her in the police station and/or an emergency department.

She broke treatment off because of persistent resistance and family criticism of residential treatment. Since then, she has had weekly psychotherapy and expressive therapy. She is confined to a single orthopaedist who is less interventionist and also has her followed up by a psychologist from his service.

Although she tries to keep herself 'straight' towards her husband, children, and the broader environment, she feels alone and abandoned. There are ongoing painful somatosensory sensations in the bikini region and other re-experiences of rape as well as haunting fears, which at times drive her to despair or suicidal ideation. Two psychotherapeutic assignments set the agenda: increased resilience so that she can free herself from her habitually meek and compliant pattern of behaviour, as well as trauma treatment, whereby this cancer can be removed, up to its furthest metastases, through psychotherapeutic microsurgery. Work on this was ongoing at the time of this writing.

## Herman—How Cain Changes into Abel

This 30-something was referred after many years of various antidepressants and psychotherapy, which had produced slight lasting improvement. Having worked as an engineer, he had been fired more than a year before. 'They didn't think I was communicative enough.' He has been suffering from feelings of rejection for about a decade. 'I have suffered from feelings of inferiority all my life.'

Herman is the eldest of three children. His younger brother is barely a year younger and is doing just fine. He is Herman's opposite. With a much younger sister, he had and has little or no connection. Father is described as a relatively calm, taciturn, contact-shy man. He is solitary and 'likes to be at ease'. Mother is willing, but he has little connection with her either. He feels that, although she asks and demands all sorts of things from him, she has little emotional availability. He always thought he should somewhat fill his father's gap. In appearance and character, he considers himself very similar to his father.

From childhood, Herman was rather shy and withdrawn. He achieved very high marks at school but had few or no friends. He could not defend himself against bullies. In college accommodation, his peers did not want to associate with him. He always felt excluded everywhere.

Over the years, the meaningful scope of an early childhood scene has become increasingly plain. After he aggressively pushed his younger brother against a cupboard, his mother went to the hospital with this bloodied sibling, and Herman was left with a neighbour. He then felt very anxious, abandoned, and punished. Since then, he has felt he had to watch meekly from his high chair as his mother lovingly cared for his younger brother.

In reality, from this incident onwards, Herman has a general aggression inhibition, whereby he allows himself to be pushed around by everyone and lets the cheese (e.g. female attention) be eaten off his bread. He cannot 'stand his ground' with either other boys or girls. He also constantly feels left out by others who get along well among themselves. He can't/doesn't dare to 'get in the middle' and thus always feels like an insignificant nobody.

First, he went through a period of several months of inpatient psychotherapy. In the group, he was timid and inhibited. He hardly ever spoke there. He behaved in a very childlike way and acted dependent towards fellow group members, but, at the same time, he had something sheepish and corny in his appearance and demeanour. This contrasted sharply with his great intelligence and high level of education.

Herman fell in love with a fellow patient who was herself very depressed, joyless, and withdrawn, not only in terms of her condition but also in terms of her character. Although he felt rejected by her, he was very submissive and clingy towards her. In variations on the theme, identification with his father and fixation on his mother were discussed at length in this context.

Fearing he would not yet be able to cope in the regular labour market, he looked for and found voluntary work in the socio-cultural sector. He was a jack-of-all-trades until he had made himself sufficiently indispensable to get a paid job. Given his degree, however, he was seriously underpaid. He gradually gained a managerial position in the operational/logistical area, but management did not fully appreciate him. Eventually, he regained full employment and a salary appropriate to his level of education . On the other hand, he continues to find it difficult to make 'real' contact with people, and certainly with women. His dealings with people are still functional. 'They never want me for who I am.' He feels loved only insofar as he is doing them a service. Also, his contacts stay fleeting and non-committal. He struggles to build a more profound and lasting bond with others. He once tested positive for being on the autism spectrum but refused to accept this (component of) diagnosis. In his feelings, childhood trauma keeps repeating itself, mainly in endless variations on the theme. He feels sidelined while others are getting along just fine and, to a greater or lesser extent, go down the intimacy route. Initially aggressively inhibited, he tries to assert himself more. Occasionally, there is an outburst of anger in which he lashes out physically. Afterwards, he feels guilty and ashamed. He also feels and/or is treated as if he has 'committed murder'. This was his feeling when his mother was gone with his little brother and left him with the neighbours. And don't you get at least life imprisonment for murder?

## Mario—Jack the (D)Ripper

Mario is a somewhat boisterous, long-haired man in his mid-30s who has already had several admissions to psychiatric hospitals, including one where he was sectioned. The latter was instituted following an incident of serious aggression towards his parents.

Mario is the eldest of five children. Father is a representative who has previously been hospitalised several times for psychiatric reasons, and there is evidence of a psychotic disorder. Mario describes him as a demanding perfectionist who finds it very difficult to express his feelings. Raised by two deaf parents and sexually abused during his teenage years, Mario's father would not have had it easy. Mario looks up to his father because of his intellect, but he does not have a good relationship with him. He was often hurt and beaten by his father. Yet there is also some sympathy and loyalty. 'Maybe he was just psychiatrically ill.'

Mother was already pregnant before marriage. Consequently, he was and felt unwanted. With her, the bond was slightly better, especially when their father was away. She had several extramarital affairs and, according to Mario, never had strong maternal feelings. He has had no contact with his parents or siblings for many years. Since he went on a rampage in their home and wrecked the place, he is afraid to meet them because he feels he is capable of murder.

Mario was brought up in an atmosphere of insecurity and tension. He was terrified, sometimes not daring to open his eyes. He was phobic of water and panicked when his hair was washed. There were many parental conflicts. His father bullied him. 'Father stood behind me when I was doing my homework, and I received a firm slap for every wrong answer.' Sometimes, his father's behaviour was strange, and he retreated to his room for several days. 'I thought he was dead.'

Mario never experienced warmth or affection; instead he received constant and arbitrary corporal punishment. From primary school age, he was severely depressed and made suicide attempts, which he said were mainly aimed at provoking parental concern. Even during this period, there was self-harm: beating the wall with his fists to the point of drawing blood or banging his knees against the ground.

During high school, he was rebellious and went down the wrong path—stealing, lying and cheating, falsifying reports, seeking out wrong friends, and running away from home. There was sexual transgressive behaviour towards one of his sisters from puberty onwards. Mother constantly promised to divorce the father but never fulfilled these words. Mario felt like a loner, depressed and misunderstood. Nowhere did he find a kind word, a hug, or comfort.

After high school, he had a lively nightlife, where he was known as a Don Juan. He has already had the most diverse jobs, including in the foreign tourism industry. 'If only I were away.' He had two long-term relationships and married his second partner. They have a baby daughter together. Because of his instability and moodiness, neither woman stayed with him.

Since the divorce, he has been squandering everything. 'I didn't care about it all anymore.' He is tired of life and feels haunted by nightmares revolving around violence, murder, and manslaughter, as well as incestuous activities where he has sex with his mother and sisters. The dreams are completely unconcealed. Drive and trauma cause total distress afterwards. He only finds solace in making metre-sized paintings in which, à la Jack—the (D)Ripper—Pollock, he goes wild with paint in an abstract, expressionist way, sometimes going beyond the limits of the canvas.

Mario was in clinical psychotherapy for several years. For a long time, he overflowed with raw and primitive emotions, mainly related to affective deficits and misdemeanours. There was a fluctuating and chaotic attachment. Sometimes, he was very positive and idealising towards the therapist; at other times, he was suspicious and hostile to the point of paranoia. He was very wild and temperamental; he needed boundaries and control to calm down and come to himself. All this also needed hefty doses of antipsychotics initially. On several occasions, he impulsively broke off his treatment and briefly went to live in remote places in various parts of the country, in search of peace and away from the others who meant hell to him. Eventually, he emigrated to a coastal village in the heel of Italy.

Since then, he has been emailing regularly and coming to consult when visiting Belgium. A solid relationship of trust has grown. He occasionally sends me a message after he learns something from his family that has upset him. This awakens his pushed-away negative feelings, quickly taking on stormy proportions without an outlet. Because I know him and his history very well, a few words that are understood are enough to calm him down, and he always responds very gratefully.

For many patients, empathic online contact can alleviate the lack of a sufficiently mirroring environmental mother in early childhood. According to Freud, civilisation began when people started hurling swear words instead of stones at each other's heads. In this sense, Mario has done a spectacular work of civilisation in his psychotherapy.

The visual work he shows also reveals this. Initially a paint-rendered chaos of drive and trauma, his work has since gained significant structure and figuration. It now refers to primitive African masks, geometric patterns, and arabesques, where primal forces are figuratively contained within a strict line formation and thus much less bursting out at the seams.

## Sam—from Whore to Madonna

Despite being in his 40s, Sam still lives with his parents. He comes in for outpatient psychotherapy because he feels something needs to change. He once lived alone for over a year but found it challenging to manage, practically and emotionally. He has been drinking excessively for about 20 years, even when he has to drive. Consequently, he has written off a car on several occasions. 'My luck will run out one day.' He worked for a company for a long time but quit owing to a lack of satisfaction. 'I expected too much: I want appreciation and impact.' Since then, he has worked as a municipal clerk. After studying classical humanities in secondary school, he obtained a bachelor's degree.

Sam is an only child. Mother is in education. She always wants to do right by everyone and is described as overprotective. *Over*protective because, sometimes, she is a bit domineering, verging on patronising. In this sense (he lets slip on acquaintance), she was, all in all, somewhat 'crippling' to his development. Father is a retired blue-collar worker. When he was little, he looked up to his father because he was so handy. Sam says he was reasonably happy for the first few years of his life. However, there were many tensions and conflicts at home owing to his father's alcohol abuse. When he had been drinking, his father was aggressive (including physically) and threatening and sometimes injured his mother, so she often had to flee the house with Sam.

Sam tried to understand and mediate, feeling constantly caught between his parents. Gradually, however, the aggression also turned against him. Now, he says of his father, 'I feel sorry for him, and I can't be angry with him anymore.' It will not change now.

He thinks his parents are making efforts but are older and weaker. He always felt different. After all, he had a secret. He had to hide something. Everything was covered up (mainly owing to pressure from his mother). After all, she insisted on keeping up appearances. For his part, Sam felt that everything was wrong at home. He never thought he belonged anywhere and anxiously tried to live up to other people's expectations. Studies came second. His main job at home was to keep and guard the peace.

Over the years, Sam has come in for outpatient psychotherapy several times. He then has about three sessions, but, each time, he breaks off treatment at this early stage. At the time of the last series of visits, he was engaged in a romantic relationship with a prostitute. Thanks to paid-for love, he had gained some sexual practice. Now he was seeing a young woman several times a week who was allegedly a victim of trafficking in women and who was reportedly terrorised by a pimp. He mainly had emotionally profound conversations with her and forged plans to rescue her from the clutches of evil men.

Although she receives him scantily clad and ready for sex, he does not need sexual contact. In contrast, an ardent platonic infatuation makes him sing of her virginal innocence, despite glaring evidence to the contrary. He has already offered her a lot of financial support and is considering kidnapping her, with all her possessions, and taking her to a safer place.

One presumably does not have to be Sigmund Freud to understand all this as an idealising maternal fixation. A romantic love purged of sensual components goes hand in hand with chivalric and rescue fantasies, eliminating the evil father/rival. Thus, Sam is among the many Oedipuses who populate the love stage.

Any attempt on my part to uncover the historical roots of this domestic drama was met with massive resistance for a long time. This otherwise intelligent man then suffered attacks of poor eyesight and hearing and repeatedly opted out of psychotherapy. Although he was very docile towards me, much-restrained anger was also palpable. He did not want to be told too much or thought having everything to say for himself was normal.

Only when his *dangerous liaison* was on the rocks and left him with a broken heart and a severely downsized wallet could he reflect on this love adventure with the necessary reflective lucidity and deduce analogies with his home situation. After many repercussions, he managed to break up with the woman. Without letting me know, he no longer turned up for his appointment. A year later, he called me, supposedly to thank me. He had since found a steady girlfriend with whom he had been for several months. He seemed incredibly proud to inform me that he would soon be getting married.

Some years later, however, he came to find me again. Apart from a brief relapse here and there, he had remained sober all this time. He still lived with his parents but, for several years, had been having an affair with a much younger female colleague he had met at work, who was also still living with her parents. They hung out a lot and also often went out or travelled. However, living together (much less getting married, cf. his earlier phone call) had never been possible. 'Neither of us were ready for it.'

His girlfriend appeared to have all kinds of fears and complexes herself. She also struggled with depression. De facto, he quickly became more of her support and advocate than her partner. He ran with her from one counselling service to another. He secured a permanent contract at work, but his boss played a 'dirty game' with him. In fact, although he had passed specific exams and was promised a promotion, a competitor landed the aspired-to post through nepotism. His girlfriend was promoted, and, although she is less qualified, her salary is now much higher than his. He has been medically signed off from work for several months owing to depression and stress and is not looking forward to returning to his workplace. 'I am seriously frustrated. Others are getting on, and I am stuck and keep tripping on the spot.'

When I ask him if the whole of the current situation with the girlfriend and the boss doesn't ring a bell with him, he immediately bursts out laughing. 'It's the same situation as at home with my parents again, surely?' Following the example of one of his friends, this time he requests admission for clinical psychotherapy himself: 'I want to get out of those patterns and change jobs'. He knows or sees that something is repeating but not yet (clearly enough) what is repeating and why. He says with a wink: 'Surely I need to analyse that further?' Without (sufficiently) doing so, that is.

## Frederik—Addicted to Abundance

This 30-something entrepreneur was referred from a rehab clinic where he had been hospitalised because of alcohol and cocaine dependence. He had also previously been hospitalised in South Africa for several months of costly rehab treatment in an exclusive residential addiction programme set up there by a private company. However, he ordered several glasses of whisky as early as when he was on the plane's return flight.

Frederik is an only child. Father combines several managerial positions in the business world. Initially, he is described as a quiet man with great ambition and commercial talents. Frederik looks up to him, has a good relationship, and speaks well with him. He does say he missed his father a lot because of his busy professional activities. Mother is described as a very dominant woman. He finds it annoying that she cannot let go of him, still wants to decide his life, and he has to toe the line. When Frederik dares to rebel, he is labelled an ungrateful child. 'That infuriates me!'

From childhood, Frederik was a cheerful, energetic, and (by his admission) 'funny' child. In primary school, he struggled with performance pressure. He changed school several times because he could not settle down. He was also bullied a lot, called a mummy's boy, laughed at, and ostracised. For high school, he was sent to a boarding school in France. It was an international crowd. He has many fond memories of the camaraderie and found much structure and support there. There were many travels during the holidays, including long-distance. He also did all sorts of activities, such as go-karting on the Azure Coast.

His university studies went awry. He sat in his digs, made no effort to study, and did nothing but go out and party. It was a lazy life of sex, drugs, and rock and roll. During that period, he says, he developed a sex addiction. There were frequent bar visits where he felt like a prince with the help of cocaine. He had sexual contact only with the most beautiful prostitutes, with photography and other models. Thanks to his father's power and influence, he was able to start a business and 'made a lot of dough' for several years.

After several years of courtship, he married a sweet, pretty, sensible girl. She was his great love. They have three children whom he says he loves to death. He hid his addiction from her. He drank secretly and snorted cocaine. When she discovered what he was doing, she initially stood beside him. Thus, she fully supported him in his detox abroad. However, when she found out that he also frequented brothels, she broke off the relationship, and a full-blown battle ensued. After that, all hell broke loose. Financial problems piled up. He had to leave and sell a lavish house, the business went bankrupt, and he hardly sees his children anymore.

Frederik was in clinical psychotherapy for several months. Superficially, he appeared to be a star pupil. He diligently participated in all therapies and activities and scored highly because of his active participation and self-critical attitude. Initially, he was an exemplary, model patient who rapidly developed various psychodynamic insights. Visibly delighted, he explained them in well-chosen terms to multiple therapists.

Soon, this turned out to be too good to be true. First, he came in dead drunk after an outing. He spent one of the following weekends snorting coke and romping with several escort women until his credit card limit was reached. Each time, he repentantly but somewhat childishly confessed his sins. However, there remained a gulf between his acceptable words and inappropriate actions for a long time.

Gradually, it became clear that the father was relatively permissive and virtually without boundaries. He took barely concealed pleasure in his son's pranks, while the mother tried to problematise her son's behaviour. In the family discussions with one of our staff, they recognised that they were de facto sponsoring his misbehaviour, and an attempt was made to minimise funding. This was not sustained for long, and, on several occasions, Frederik and his children were taken to luxurious and exotic holiday destinations.

It took a lot for Frederik to realise that he was addicted to a horn of plenty. Once we agreed on this, a change began. Of course, it was no mean feat for him to abstain from all sorts of pleasures. After all, it is not easy to voluntarily leave a *Playboy* mansion to earn a hard living by the sweat of one's brow. It took a laborious process to reconcile with the necessary mortifications.

As is well known, there are very different conceptions, as well as manifestations, of narcissistic personality disorders. In some, it is a developmental disorder, where (classically Freudian) there is a fixation on His Majesty the Baby's oral and narcissistic gratifications. In others, narcissism is a defensive bastion against oral and narcissistic deprivation.

In the first case, empathic mirroring and dosed frustration will be central to the technique. In the second, mentalisation-promoting therapy and/or interpretation of negative (transference) feelings will mostly be in the foreground.

Frederik belonged to the first category. Only after much falling (into substance use) and getting up did he achieve total abstinence. He now lives in a modest flat and, for now, finds contentment in employment. We have patiently continued mirroring and mentalising his ups and downs on good and bad days. In clinical practice, this always bears more fruit than all kinds of attempts at correction.

## Gerard—Entre-Deux-Mères

This young 40-something was referred to a PWGH service because of a crisis he cannot get out of.

> I was panicking, at my wit's end, seeing no way out. My life became a soup. I was torn apart. Sofie, my ex-wife, was the love of my life. We got married on our 21st and divorced two years later. But we always kept in touch. We were jealous of each other's lives. We are both in different relationships that we question. I kept dreaming of Sofie and fantasising about her. I was never able or willing to let her go. I always cherished the thought that one day things would work out. Then, after twenty years, I found the courage to talk about my lingering feelings. We went into our love, and I lived a double life for several months. Until I confessed everything to Sylvie, my current wife. I felt remorse. She also started noticing that something was wrong. Now, I can't say we are just moving on.

Gerard has been married to Sylvie, a healthcare worker, for about 20 years. They have two sons. Sofie was his first steady sweetheart. He met her when he was 16. He found in her the warmth he missed at home. 'I am a small wagon, not a locomotive.'

Gerard's parents were self-employed and had little or no time for him. Their bakery opened a week after he was born and wholly absorbed them. For high school, he was sent to boarding school. It was a large institution where the law of the jungle prevailed and where he struggled to stand his ground because of his small stature. He wept a lot there. During weekends, he had to help full-time in the business. Often, he longed to break out.

Sofie also came from a home with little warmth. She had 'no emotional bond' with her parents. In no time, they became deeply attached. After two years of marriage, they went on an exotic group trip with peers. There, a world opened up for Sofie. They were all singles or young couples enjoying life to the fullest. She felt she had missed something and fell in love with another boy. 'However, he was a real adventurer.' This break-up caused Gerard considerable hurt. Sofie later married another man and had two adolescent children. She is currently divorcing and has bought a new home.

Gerard feels the bond with his parents has dramatically improved since they stopped their business. Mother now feels guilty that she has not been there enough for him. His parents were both busy with the bakery 24/7. There was no room for a family or social life. Moreover, father went to the pub after work. 'He fled the house.' Consequently, the mother was often alone with her children. 'She grieved a lot. She sought company, support and warmth from us.' As a result of various unclear health problems, she also needed a lot of help and care.

Feeling unbearable guilt, Gerard confessed to his wife. People often want to free themselves from unbearable distress caused by their conscience by exposing their hearts and souls to the wrong person. They then 'confess to the devil', as it were. Freud once called psychoanalysis a confession without absolution. Indeed, his consulting room is a better-suited space to scrutinise sometimes violently conflicting feelings, expose their roots, and help people make conscious ethical choices. In the process, they are not unquestioningly guided by some gospel but seek to find/invent their own authentic answer to essentially unanswerable questions. Mother, why do we live? What does it mean to be a man or a woman? What is happiness? What makes a fulfilling partner relationship? What is the basis of law or authority? What are we talking about when we talk about love?

Countless times, Gerard compared the two women. He listed their qualities and flaws. What attracted and repelled him? He tried to suppress, reason away, or distract his feelings. All this did not change his primordial attachment to his first love. For him, she has something that cannot be imagined or put into words—something Gerard does not have (any more), which he misses and longs for. A desire without reason(s) imposes its will on him. It is as in Bizet's opera *Carmen*: '*L'amour est un oiseau rebelle qui n'a jamais connu de loi*'. Love is a rebellious bird that has never known any law. Unless it is what Jacques Lacan calls the law of the Thing: that original some Thing we lost after separation from the mother and for which we nostalgically yearn in an attempt to find it (again). It is a Thing that imposes its will or whim on us.

Although he cannot understand, argue with, or motivate it, Gerard goes for *it* and, in the process and for that, leaves behind everything he has. He does not recognise himself in the steps he takes while sensing he is being true to his most intimate core and deepest being. It makes his choice an authentic act, abandoning societal convention in saying 'yes' to the Thing.

Throughout this decision, Gerard feels at once more than ever strange and more than ever himself. It causes much heartache, as he feels a devoted love for both mothers and wives, whom—albeit for different reasons—he values sincerely and highly. At the same time, his choice brings about a radical individuation and separation, and he only really feels separated by his divorce. Only now, he feels better able to act as a more sovereign and autonomous locomotive for his newly reconstituted family.

## Linda—the Ugly Duckling

This woman, in her 40s, seems hidden behind a curtain of hair. With her angry eyes, it is as if she is watching me from a hidden position in the bushes. She begins by saying that she feels empty, lifeless, and irritable. She has been hospitalised elsewhere several times for this. It is said to have worsened, especially after the death of her father two years before. He was a blue-collar and 'diligent' worker. He would have been helpful, but he was short-tempered, and Linda feared him. His will was, after all, law. Still, she knew he loved her very much. Mother is considered a problematic woman. She is resentful and is 'as stubborn as a mule'.

Linda still lives at home, mainly for financial reasons. She works part-time in the care sector. In terms of relationships, she had an affair with a slightly older man who, however, did not want to commit. She only really fell in love with a German man she had met online. They were constantly webcamming for several months. He asked her to do all kinds of sexual things. For instance, she had to undress in front of the camera and masturbate, and, when they met in the flesh, they were soon playing BDSM games. She allowed all this to happen because she was in love with him. However, after he broke off the relationship, she felt abused and cheated. She also lent him a lot of money that she never got back. Despite all these negative feelings, she misses the attention and love she received from him.

From childhood, Linda was very embarrassed, shy, and insecure. She was bullied and humiliated throughout primary and secondary school because of her chunky and somewhat masculine appearance. She always put up with it but, on the other hand, stood up for the underdog. Despite everything, the 'relationship' with the German was, therefore, an emotional and sexual revelation for her. For the first time, she felt like number 1 instead of number 13,972 (a number she often, bitterly, used for herself). She also felt coveted and (literally and figuratively) liked, even in her naked state.

She was in inpatient psychotherapy for about a year. There were persistent narcissistic problems: she had a very low and fragile self-image, especially as a woman. She also had great difficulty expressing her feelings, and she needed to make copious use of all kinds of collages she made in expressive therapy. I liken it to dreaming by proxy. Patients are invited to cut out images and words from magazines that *tell* them something about all sorts of psychosexual and social themes, often without their knowing (exactly) what. In conversations, they are then asked to express free thoughts about the various fragments that map their inner world with the help of the therapist.

With Linda, two themes prevailed. She always puts herself in an 'ASO' position (her term)—at the service of ... In this way, she tries to earn love and attention, which, she feels, never come spontaneously or unconditionally. She gradually built more self-confidence and self-love thanks to consistent mirroring of her insides and self-image. This became clear in her appearance as she became more coquettish, changed her hairstyle, and started using lipstick and mascara for the first time.

She still regularly falls back into a (too) compliant, obliging, or user-friendly attitude, but she recognises this automatism and tries to adjust, with varying success. From a grown 'basic trust', she can and dares express all kinds of complaints and dissatisfactions, making her more assertive and resilient in conflicts with others.

## Bernard—She Matters

Bernard is 40-something and has been attending weekly psychotherapy for about five years. His first words:

> I am getting nowhere with studies or work. Relationships are difficult. My head has trouble keeping up with my heart. I fall in love too easily. The problem was acute many years ago. I met a woman who had just come out of a relationship. I didn't know that. She did not want an intimate relationship with me. She was emotionally unavailable. I knew it wouldn't be anything, but I couldn't disengage.

He is the middle of three sons. The father was an officer in the Air Force, and the mother was a housewife. At home, he felt he fell a bit between two seats. 'I was not taken seriously.' He once told his mother he wanted to be a pilot as a boy. She ridiculed this dream. One word he uses for her in the intake interview is 'einschränkend' (belittling). In the sessions, he often abandons his mother tongue and switches to English or German. He further calls her overprotective, condescending, narrow-minded. 'I could do nothing right for her.'

His father he describes as restrained and disciplined. He was the authority in the house. 'Be a man!' was his motto. Before him, a child had died. It is never spoken of. He never felt very much at home. 'Like I was irrelevant.' Street and school were also quite unfriendly to him. Peers often bullied him, and, under the slogan 'Not with me', he turned away from humanity early on. He dropped out of several university courses. Not because of poor results, as he got excellent marks in many subjects, but because he did not like 'the system'. Eventually, the university authorities did not allow him to continue his studies.

In his primary school days, a girl lived across the street. She often sat behind the window on the first floor, smiling sweetly whenever she saw him, giving him a warm feeling. During therapy, it becomes increasingly clear that this young woman (whom he called his Mona Lisa at one point) set the tone.

For instance, he is an avid photographer. He is often on the lookout for models—not for glamour, fashion, or erotic photos, but for an ideal image that he seems to have in mind that he tries to realise with the cooperation of the women concerned. He puts great effort into these photo shoots. He does not even shy away from travelling to another country. However, he does nothing with the photographs—at least, nothing profitable. They only play a role in his *inner* economy.

I gave the word 'icon' to him for such images. I naturally thought of icons from the Greek Orthodox Church, particularly images of the Madonna and Child. I also often thought of the feature film *Et Dieu créa la femme* (And God Created Woman) or the Pygmalion theme exploited by Irish playwright George Bernard Shaw that later became known to the broader public through the blockbuster *My Fair Lady*. In them, the artist falls in love with his created image.

Bernard talks a lot about whether or not he has '*rapport*' (French) with his environment. He notes that he can feel *rapport* not only with other people but also with specific things. Why does one person or travel destination appeal to him more than another? What is he looking for? It turns out, more than once, that he does not want to get away but, on the contrary, wants to feel at home somewhere.

Currently, he lives mainly from translation work. He works for companies and sometimes has to do final editing. He is meticulous and annoyed by the disregard of other or earlier translators. He makes it a point of honour to find the *right* word to meet a standard he sets for himself. He can sometimes spend a whole day brooding on a word. His price per word is comparable to that of other translators, but, when he calculates how much he earns per hour, he turns out to toil for a pittance. Moreover, his meticulous perfectionism often leads to him working at night so that he can meet deadlines. On the other hand, he does like working when everyone else is asleep. It gives him a sense of freedom.

One of the subjects he tried was mathematics. He likes its purity. He also plays with the literal meaning (in Dutch, mathematics is '*wis-kunde*'—literally, the art of erasure). He is then concerned with erasing negative mirroring that he constantly experienced because of his mother.

I remind him of an anecdote from when he was on a class trip to the Alps. Everyone was nattering, laughing, and joking on a terrace. He left the group to enjoy the cold mountain air and snow-capped peaks. He talks about his abstract thinking but thinks the word abstract is not well chosen. I juxtapose the words 'ideas' and 'ideals' for him (not for the first time).

Then, he suddenly says he is thinking of Julie, with whom he recently did a photo shoot. He does not understand why he is thinking about her. There is *something* about her, but he can't say what. He doesn't find her sexually attractive, but there's something about her eyes. Or with eye contact. However, he adds that eye contact also has much to do with the rest of the facial expression. One thing is for sure: she *matters*! With my free-floating attention, I hear these two words obliquely, with the emphasis not on the second word but on the first. *She* matters. That Bernard struggles with She matters is, indeed, a hard fact.

The next time, he had to cancel because of the funeral of his elder brother. He begins by saying: 'I should have been in Vienna'. A photography exhibition was taking place there, which he had reluctantly had to miss. He would also have gone there to see works by Klimt. In his young adulthood, he had a fierce but unrequited infatuation with Leen. She gave him only one thing as a gift: a card by Klimt. I remember the words 'she was just coming out of a relationship' chiming with the mother having lost a child before him. I invite him to elaborate a bit more on this love story.

Bernard lay awake for several days before daring to express his feelings to her. He immediately had a hunch that it would end unhappily, but he did not believe in it. He then talked about his *Weltanschauung*, which is all about unrequited and impossible love. Hie father was absent; in his mother's eyes, he was always wrong. He felt he didn't belong at home.

He felt like a '*quantité négligeable*' (negligible quantity), not only to his parents but also to his brothers. His aloof and (nicely put) 'reserved' attitude towards fellow (predominantly female) humans is a fatal defence mechanism against rejection. Fateful because it functions as a self-fulfilling prophecy. 'It's all good to understand how I get to it, but how to break this automatism?'

We have been working on this task for several years. His progress in doing so is remarkable. He starts associating in response to this or that detail but often stays in stratospheres. He exhausts himself in all sorts of theoretical reflections on his problems and only after my repeated prompting does he produce raw, empirical data from his childhood and youth. In doing so, he keeps returning to his toddler years, when a stubborn and unyielding 'no' to his mother installed itself and where he wanted to be guided only by his firmness of principle. It made for a monotonous and socially isolated stereotype only occasionally punctuated by international escapades to a hoped-for (because it was perceived to be a more hospitable) motherland.

## Christiane—through a Valley of Tears

This 50-year-old woman had already been hospitalised in a PWGH service three times for depressive symptoms. At her mother's birthday party, she crashed again. Her favourite brother was present with a new partner, over 20 years younger. 'I can't process it. It's like he's making love to his child.' In other words, the word 'incest' can be read between the lines at once. Another brother has gone totally off the rails and is serving a prison sentence of years for violent theft. Christiane can't stand her mother's worries either. It all becomes too much and too powerful for her.

Christiane is the second of three children. Her father died when she was an adolescent. He had alcoholism and, under the influence of alcohol, was physically aggressive towards his wife and children, who regularly had to flee to various neighbours. Christiane would then crawl into a corner somewhere and wet herself in terror. Occasionally, there was sexually transgressive behaviour towards her. The mother is described as mentally strong. After all, she had endured all the difficulties with her father. On the other hand, she was not home much because she was at work a lot.

Early on, Christiane took on many care duties as an only daughter. She tried to be good and brave and was very concerned about the ups and downs of the others. Both brothers fought regularly. Christiane always tried to mediate. She found it hard to shut herself off from other people's problems: 'I'm like a sponge.' After a technical education, she worked as a textile worker for a long time. She is happily married and has two children with no apparent problems.

Christiane underwent three admissions, with several months of clinical psychotherapy with us each time. During these treatment episodes, there was sometimes severe regression, during which she appealed for help a lot, as she needed maternal care. There were constantly triggers for post-traumatic relapses related to violence and incestuous transgressive behaviour on the part of the father.

For a long time, a torrent of tears was the only outlet for all her emotional content. She learned to differentiate her emotional world better through our providing the necessary mentalising development aid. In particular, she had much trouble mobilising 'healthy aggression' when it came to conflicts with her brother (they were like 'two peas in a pod'), for instance.

Between and after admissions, she was and is in weekly psychotherapy. A marriage in which she lived as brother and sister with her husband for decades finds an entirely new, erotic character. This patient's highly dependent and childlike-to-tame attitude provokes much countertransference paternalism. Because she was taken seriously and her feelings and story were listened to thoughtfully, emancipatory forces were awakened in her that no one from her environment had thought possible.

## Andre—Hello, Strange Man

When asked to 'tell me', Andre replied, broadly, as follows:

> I have had problems since childhood. I was bullied in primary school. My parents took me to a child psychiatrist. She gave me medication for motor disorders. I also went to a physiotherapist for a long time. When I was sixteen, a psychologist discovered that I was homosexual. I have trouble just accepting that. I do find it hard to become independent from home. Over a year ago, I had a panic attack. I then started scratching my head and attempted suicide with pills. I was hospitalised at a

psychotherapy centre for five months. Afterwards, I started working in counselling. I have also had an urge to visit gay car parks and gay saunas for years. I am wrung with that. Since my second suicide attempt earlier this year, I have been doing voluntary work in the LGBTQIA+ sector.

Initially, Andre says he has a good relationship with his parents. In particular, he says he is very attached to his mother, with whom, after all, he would always find comfort and security and from whom he finds it hard to be apart. He describes her as concerned but says she is also dominant and short-tempered. Father is described as quiet, withdrawn, and absent. He can be very controlling, however. He is said to have difficulty dealing with emotions. Andre has an older brother whom he describes as very compulsive. His mother would have been scared at the time of Andre's birth. Her mother had died a year before. 'I think I already felt as a baby that my mum was anxious.'

By his admission, he was always a problematic child, wanting to have his say and play boss. There was much bickering and/or competition with his older brother. 'Who is number 1?' In his preschool years, he mainly played with girls. There was only one African boy with whom he got along well. In one of the later conversations, the phrase 'woman is the nigger of the world' escaped him in this context.

Andre struggled to stand his ground; he tried to stay home by shouting, ranting, crying, or even hiding in the toilet. At school, he was called a 'sissy'; he felt unaccepted and rejected. In adolescence, he met with his mother instead of going out. He would never have been rebellious, was in bed a lot, and had problems with his homosexual orientation. Apart from alternating and short-term contacts, he was in a steady relationship for two years and lived with Simon, who was a few years older.

In the second conversation, Andre talked about how difficult it was to get close to his father. He never felt comfortable with him. 'Actually, I don't know my father.' He immediately recounted two dreams. He had dreamed that he tried to explain to his father that going to gay car parks or saunas was no big deal. That it was a natural need. In his dream, he started weeping and thought of suicide. He was afraid his father wouldn't take his story seriously or would deny it.

In a connecting dream, he dreamed he was having sex with his older brother. He was licking his toes, moving slowly up his legs. He woke up with an incredibly foul and sour taste in his mouth. The subsequent associations were about him feeling neither supported nor affirmed by his father. Licking his toes reminded him of his slavish or canine submission—the sour taste of the trouble he had with what he called his homosexual excesses.

In the next session, he said he had never learned to deal with his drives. He said he had a strong maternal bond, was a sickly, worried child, and was always exemplary, reasonable, and considerate. In retrospect, he also considered himself overly religious. He said Hail Marys daily and read the Bible.

He then followed with stories of how he was overwhelmed by his mother's love and closeness. 'Mother sought comfort from me. I was her friend.'

Other mother figures in the family also took excessive care of him. At the same time, there was father hunger. 'I am constantly seeking a man to set boundaries and bring clarity. However, one man would not be enough. I would want all the men in the world.' One of his favourite songs of the time was 'Hello, Strange Man' by the late Flemish singer An Christy. Andre experiences a great desire for sex. He masturbates several times a day. He fantasises about the men he meets. 'We look at each other like two hot dogs.'

He talks about his doubts. Am I more likely to be male or more likely to be female? Am I attracted to men or women? He sees his homosexual acting-out behaviour as evacuating and venting mostly aggressive tensions and frustrations. It is a complex action symptom in which he greedily searches for the phallus he wants to eat and absorb, but in which he also actively controls and can express a 'fuck you' feeling. In this context, he recounts a dream in which he shits on a Mercedes. Since his father is a car mechanic, Andre calls cars 'sacred cows'. The aggressive part of his homosexual behaviour is thus unmistakable, which does not mean that Andre does not repeatedly forget these and other unconscious determinants. Repression is a nasty beast.

Andre was in inpatient psychotherapy for about a year. Afterwards, he came for weekly outpatient group psychotherapy for two years and has been coming for weekly face-to-face individual psychotherapy for about ten years. He went through a very significant evolution. Initially, all the aggression had a frightening and disruptive effect on him. His parents were getting on his nerves, literally and figuratively—his mother by her patronising and, therefore, emasculating attitude, and his father by his absence, his denigrating attitude towards women and femininity, and his flurry of implicitly belittling bemusement. In countless variations on the theme, it was about the good and generous Andre trying to push away and swallow up all phallic rebellion and defiance. The result was free-floating anxiety and panic attacks and, as a barometer of his tension level, homosexual acting-out behaviour to let off steam.

He has been in a steady relationship for ten years, living with a slightly older girlfriend he has known since college. Because of fertility problems on his part, they turned to adoption after unsuccessful infertility treatments. Andre is a devoted father who takes his only son's psychosexual development very seriously. He runs his own designer goods business and has been self-employed for years. He works hard to keep his head above water and his parents out of it. His increasing empowerment towards customers and suppliers goes hand in hand with a steady decline in his sauna visits.

Conversely, for him, the latter urge is an extremely sensitive and reliable indicator of all kinds of things that 'bother' him. He invented a new term for this symptom—'*phallophilia*'. The end of his psychotherapy is not yet in sight. He appreciates further psychological counselling for the time being. While he initially consumed an impressive cocktail of atypical antipsychotics, antidepressants, and anxiolytics, he has been doing without pharmacotherapy entirely in recent years. 'That's the most important thing, because with psychotherapy—however long—I don't hurt anyone.'

## Trui—Late Birth

This woman, who is in her early 30s, was referred from a PWGH service where she was first hospitalised. Her opening words: 'I don't know who I am or what I want. Or I might know, but I don't *want* to know'. It's all hard to explain, according to her. She feels like she is in a whirlpool, not knowing which door to take. 'What is the right choice?' On closer inspection, this impasse has always been there. At most, there were periods of pause. Even when she was young, the question, 'What is the point?' overwhelmed her. At 18, she took an overdose of medication for the first time. She then 'started cutting to avoid crying'.

For a while, she wrote poems and then said to herself, 'Stop doing that. Act normal'. Trui met her husband when she was 19 and married him after a five-year courtship. They have two children, but she says she barely has maternal feelings. 'I always said I didn't want to have children. They weep. They are troublesome. I have no patience for all that.' The spouses live side by side. He has his own business and, therefore, he is there and he is not there. Only work seems to count.

Trui is the eldest of five children, and they all help in the parental business. Her mother is a housewife. She is 'ordinary'. 'She says she works a lot, but I wonder what she does.' She finds her mother rather lazy and sloppy. 'Superficially', they get along well. Her father is a hard worker and, therefore, never at home. He is also very closed-minded. Trui constantly feels that he is disappointed in her. 'He will say it's not true, but I still feel that way.' At school, Trui was bullied a lot. 'We weren't good enough.' She never felt she belonged anywhere. Also, the fact that she could not write without mistakes led to her being laughed at for perceived stupidity. She was later found to have dyslexia, but people did not want to hear or see this.

Especially from high school onwards, there was a great sense of failure. She took refuge in reading during her adolescence, especially *fantasy* stories with their world of elves and dragons. She also started going out and then hung out with 'the tough ones' by drinking a lot, being defiant to boys, and being out of control on the dance floor. She has been smoking in secret since she was 14, but no one around her knows anything about it. Earlier in the year, she met another man through social media whom she had dated and kissed several times. Partly because of this, she is baffled and lost her head.

Superficially, this woman has always functioned 'normally'. She has always kept up with the rest and the pace of life. At the same time, she is almost existentially frustrated and lacks meaning. 'Mother, why are we living?'

'There is something here inside' is a quote from a once-popular pop song that used to appeal to her. She knows there is something but not *what* there is.

She has yet to be psychically born, as it were. Our insides unfold only to the extent that they are mirrored and acknowledged by parents. In the absence of such emotional attunement, Trui was left saddled with a pack of untold and, over time, unbearable feelings. She is randomly searching for life experiences that *tell* her something.

She was in clinical psychotherapy for six months. The patient is offered an artificial environment where the average temperature, understanding, emotional support, and empathy are much higher than in the natural one. In Donald Winnicott's terms, this is a holding and facilitating maternal environment. Our team sometimes speaks of enriched potting soil in which even the saddest plant can be brought to unexpected growth and flowering.

An intensive therapy programme is, then, likened to a menu. It provides balanced nutrition. By analogy, fats, carbohydrates, proteins, vitamins, and so on are fundamentally of equal importance. Of course, some are found to be more palatable than others, but all therapies and activities are offered as a kind of *work*. Each patient will deal with them in highly individual ways. Possibilities, talents, problems, and resistances are made noticeable and discussable. Thus, people get to know the most diverse sides of themselves. All the more so because, at each stumbling block, they are invited to tell something about their history.

Classically, psychoanalytic therapy is called insight-giving. However, gaining insight into problems' origins and persistence is only one therapeutic factor. Psychotherapy does not only involve clarifying mental contents. It also implies a form of developmental aid stimulating mental processes. After admission, Trui did another year of outpatient psychotherapy with a psychologist combined with monthly psychiatric and psychoanalytic process counselling with me. So many years later, she still comes several times a year. She insists on continuing to share her life's journey with me. Please don't ask her to explain precisely what has changed with her. 'I can only say that my life has only started since admission.'

## Lutgard—First on the Road, Then on Her Way

This 30-year-old woman was referred from a PWGH where she had not got out of a slump despite multiple hospital admissions.

> I struggle with the past. I can't process it. I went through something. I had to stand on my own two feet from age eighteen. I was pushed backwards by my siblings. Father never worked. He is at the sick bay. He was lying on the couch, and he had to be served. My eldest sister and I had to work, work, work. I went babysitting a lot to get away from home. From the age of fourteen, I did apprenticeships. I always had to hand over all my money. My parents sat on the sofa with their hands open. Father was aggressive towards us: hitting us, dragging us down the stairs by the hair,

literally putting the knife to our throats, hurling an iron at our heads. He also sexually abused me between the ages of twelve and eighteen. Then I ran away from home.

Lutgard is the second of four children. Her father is a blue-collar worker. She calls him a psychopath. According to her, he is a hypocritical liar. He was vicious, controlling, and constantly menacing. He constantly belittled Lutgard. He called her an ugly duckling, '*kwek kwek kwek kwek*'. Her mother is described as naive and not too sensible. She goes about her business. She may mean well, but she is unreliable and does not see things as they are. She has betrayed Lutgard's trust many times.

Since childhood, Lutgard has been anxious and insecure. She was bullied a lot at school. Students spat on her because she was supposedly not one of the brightest. She still found some happiness in the youth movement. She was allowed to travel with friends' parents; these were her best times. She was also often cared for at her aunt and uncle's house. Her cousin felt like a real sister.

She always hid and concealed everything. She withdrew into her shell. The family fell apart after her parents' divorce (when she was 19). She hardly saw her siblings anymore. However, their father kept harassing her, picking fights, and making death threats. She does not know where he lives but feels unsafe to this day. She has never had a real relationship. She struggles with intimacy and sexuality.

She works in a shop and moonlights in catering at night and at weekends. This allows her to avoid standing still and having to think. After the suicide of a bosom friend, her isolation and loneliness have become unbearable.

Innumerable patients 'enter psychiatry' with a similar history. Often, the help they receive is symptom-focused—a prescription for medication—and/or solution-focused—supportive and essentially covering up (i.e. a recovery instead of a discovery approach). In this way, they try to ensure that they can cope. Often, this leads to a dumbing down, with increasingly dire consequences for relationships and socio-professional engagements. This inevitably results in increasing marginalisation and/or disablement. Indeed, there is a prognostically fatal combination of deficits in basic security/nurturing and (in this case, sexual) trauma.

A more fundamental and lasting remedy is possible only when work is done to build a robust therapeutic relationship. Within this, both mentalisation and a corrective emotional experience can take place. A digestive process also needs to be started. Post-traumatic symptoms can broadly be understood as regurgitations of what remains raw and undigested in the stomach. Through chewing and rumination (by both patient and therapist), many words and saliva must be used to make them sink in sufficiently. Only then do regurgitations (flashbacks, somatosensory sensations, nightmares) diminish, and the traumatic experiences 'take their place' without, however, ever disappearing entirely from the patient's memory or recollection.

Lutgard required a one-and-a-half-year admission, first in full-time hospitalisation, then in day treatment, and then in part-time treatment (several half-days a week). This was combined with assisted living and the partly overlapping start of outpatient therapy. It was a process with a lot of ups and downs on her part and holding on and letting go on our part. In the meantime, she finished care training, is working as a carer, and is preparing to live independently. She feels 'on her way' instead of 'on the road'—an essential difference many patients testify to after a somewhat long journey.

## Kyara—an Alley Cat

Kyara is a swaggering, boyish-presenting adolescent who has already had several juvenile psychiatric admissions. She now requests further inpatient psychotherapy herself. 'I have wanted to put everything away. I don't want to talk about it. My brother died. I miss him. Several mates have committed suicide. It's all become too much.'

Kyara is the youngest of four children. Her favourite brother died in a crash when she was 16. They were very close and were real 'buddies'. Kyara was always with him. They could go to each other for anything and everything. She misses him immensely. Her parents divorced when she was 12. There was a lot of turmoil at home. The children were often beaten by both parents. She always felt abandoned at home. Since then, she has lived with her father. She was his darling. She describes him as a rough husk with a soft heart. He is closed, raw, and brutal in his dealings. 'With his drunken bollocks, he spits everything out.' She likes him but does not get on well with her stepmother.

She feels neither understood nor believed by her mother. 'She hurt me a lot.' Kyara pictures her as very selfish and dramatising. It's always 'Me, me, me'. On the one hand, she makes a mountain out of a molehill while, on the other hand, she doesn't take things that matter seriously. She mainly retains this feeling from being sexually abused by a friend of her sister. It almost came to rape, but fortunately someone intervened. After a brother read diary excerpts, the police got involved. However, her mother never really believed her. After this abuse, she started self-harming. The trauma is still very haunting and has barely been digested.

Kyara was a real tearaway. She often ran away from home and was like a bad boy who did a lot of mischief. She felt better on the streets than at home. With tears in her eyes, she says you always have to return home in the end. Because of all the mess and misery at home, she could sometimes get very frustrated, hitting the wall with her fists or 'starting to break down the shack' in her room. At school, she had some trouble with authority. 'I didn't like being told anything.' She was sociable and had many boyfriends and girlfriends. At 15, she had her first relationship, with a boy three years her senior, who tamed her somewhat 'because I was a wild one!'

Time and patience are indispensable in any psychotherapy. At the time of this writing, Kyara has been in psychotherapy almost continuously for a decade, with prolonged episodes of day hospitalisation and shorter ones in between on an outpatient basis. She was very volatile for many years—almost daily cannabis use, countless fugues, and unauthorised absences. She did have a steady cohabiting relationship with a peer for many years. They stayed together after many good but also bad days.

She also remained 'loyal' to our hospital, where she took part in successive inpatient psychotherapy within the youth, young adult, and adult care programmes. She always presented as very tough and angry. She looked like Eminem for a long time, with a hoodie, headphones, heavy hiking boots, and so on. In recent years, she has sometimes dressed very femininely and even sexily, with a fashionable hairstyle, Wonderbra, and bare legs.

Her cannabis use has stopped, and the fugues have stopped. Changes include the externalisation of a more secure attachment system with spectacularly increased mentalising ability and a stable and greatly more positive self-image as a woman.

Currently, she is going into detail about all sorts of things, including about her completely unaligned mother who, after all, did not mirror her or mirrored her wrongly. She was regularly slapped by her and penetrated by her on occasion for insertion of suppositories and lavages up to a far too advanced (primary school) age. There were many fights involving physical violence at home, which made her feel almost like a war child. This was clear in numerous dreams where she found herself in a guerrilla or civil war where the enemy invaded her home, and she was not safe there. On the streets, she was at the mercy of (equally dissolute) homeless lowlifes who grew up without god or commandment, used drugs, and indulged sexual urges (including on her). Thus, she was not only a victim of sexual abuse perpetrated by a friend of her sister's, and, gradually, more re-experiences appeared of a situation where she felt almost literally caged and had to endure a gang rape.

Wouldn't you later run at the slightest sense of deprivation of liberty that inevitably accompanies any therapy situation and relationship? Since initially not only her Ego but also her Superego was very unintegrated, she also got into fringe criminal activities (dealing, etc.). She did run away from the truth more often than not, not only because of the long duration of her treatment or the persistence of her acting-out behaviour but also because of her 'dishonesty'; many feelings of rejection by team members had to be contained and interpreted.

Eventually, we opted for weekly outpatient psychotherapy. The foundations of a trusting relationship had been sufficiently well established. Her acting-out style and difficulty with laws and rules (which she continued to experience as a form of power or coercion for the time being) led to all sorts of rearguard actions, which sometimes hindered rather than eased the actual psychotherapeutic process. She shows up punctually and produces free association and dream material revolving around abandonment and trauma. She still often finds herself in dubious environments and marginal situations, but somehow manages to keep her 'cool' and poise there. It is clear, though, that she does not let anything or anyone get her down. The most significant difficulty she still has is with her soft side/feelings. She is terrified of being passive and resists this danger like a devil in a basin of holy water.

After all these years, she dares to cry now and then to show her sadness or affection, proving that a lot has already changed in her attachment system. She is now fully engaged in clearing her sexual feelings. Meanwhile, she has a real mother–child relationship with her partner. She speaks baby language and allows herself to be cherished and cuddled by her friend, but there is no sign of libido towards her.

Her erotic fantasies revolve around a negatively Oedipal constellation, in which she sexually *shows* older, but (in her eyes) also sexy and classy, women 'every corner of the room'. In doing so, she visibly enjoys poking fun at male pirates. On the other hand, there is also a passive–active reversal, where she holds power and revels in her potency. Through erotic party games, she tries to rekindle the fire in her partner's relationship while scrutinising and working on her feelings of attraction and repulsion in psychotherapy. After all, she wants to build a stable partner relationship.

At the time of this writing, she seems to have given up this 'battle'. The couple no longer live as mother and son but as brother and sister—that is, on a more equal footing. They do many fun and friendly things together, but sex and romance seem well and truly out of the question for Kyara from now on. She does not want to indulge in sexual escapades (she fantasises about going to a brothel). 'I don't dare.' Fantasy may remain a fantasy for her. The reality and stability of her relationship are too precious to her.

## Myriam—a Quick Fix

Myriam is a brightly made-up young woman living with a peer who has worked as a clerk for several years. She works in the care sector but, for the past three years, she has been at home on sick pay because of depressive symptoms, head and muscle pains, nausea, and inner turmoil. She was referred for inpatient psychotherapy by her GP. By her own account, she thinks a lot. Father was a heavy alcoholic and violent when he drank. Her parents are divorced, and her mother lives with her current boyfriend, who is also said to be an alcoholic and physically aggressive.

Myriam is the younger of two daughters. Her sister claims to have no problems. From childhood, Myriam felt left out partly because she was on the obese side. She got by with her big mouth and felt better at school than at home. She has always been terrified but managed to hide this from everyone. She has had no contact with her father for years. He was a police officer who brought his service weapon home and constantly threatened to use it when specific things did not suit him. Myriam appeared to be his darling, which meant she suffered less from his misbehaviour than her mother and sister.

'It's all very confusing; I was a spectator and a victim. I put on a big mouth against Father, but on the other hand, I also proved him right.' She knew how to appease and/or win him over. Her mother is a teacher and also works as a secretary. 'I don't know what kind of person my mother is. But she must be strong; otherwise, she wouldn't have lasted fifteen years with my father.' It was forbidden to talk about the misery at home, though, because of Mother; everything had to stay hidden. 'All my life, I have been seeking acknowledgement and validation from her, but she refuses to talk about the past.'

Myriam has been in clinical psychotherapy with us for barely six months. She could tell her story for the first time and felt acknowledged and understood. We talked most extensively about her habitual tendency to erotically charm men. This originated as a kind of Stockholm syndrome where hostages join or even fall in love with their captors out of self-defence and an attempt at life preservation. Above all, she found peace and security with us, especially as she entered a relationship with a rather meek and completely non-violent young man and fellow group member. Both found a lot of care and nurturing in this relationship, and so their problems seemed 'solved'.

If one of them had to end clinical psychotherapy with us after first her and later his discharge from our hospital, it came down to Myriam managing everything. She worked full-time, caring for the household and her new 'off-spring'. Thanks to all this, she felt like lord and master. Therefore, she had 'everything under control' and only sporadically visited the psychologist.

I saw her several more times, monthly. She could then clearly see that, with this relationship, under the form of enactment, she was satisfying a repressed need. After all, she lovingly fathered and mothered a youngster whom she considered a (similarly) small and helpless other-equal. Meanwhile, she knew all too well that she was running from actual therapy, but, thanks to her busy schedule, she hardly had time to dwell on herself and her feelings. She realises this will turn sour sooner or later, but, 'As long as it lasts, I try to go at it full steam ahead'. She asked for an appointment via email twice afterwards but did not reply to my emails when I suggested a concrete time to her.

A few years later, she came for a consultation. She had undergone gastric bypass surgery and was almost unrecognisable because she had turned into a kind of vamp. For her, her sexy potency is a tool of choice to play men. In the process, she experiences power and control, which she enjoys on the one hand but describes as illusory on the other. However masterfully she plays the erotic register, she lacks a sufficiently secure foundation. Hopefully, she will soon find her way back to further psychotherapy.

## Iris—Daughter, Mother, Wife

This 30-year-old woman was referred for outpatient psychotherapy by a fellow psychiatrist. 'I am scared of my thoughts. It started about three years ago after the birth of my eldest daughter. I see images of children getting sick and dying.' She continues:

My mother had a heart attack in [three years before]. Initially, I tried to cut these weird thoughts by thinking of other things. Fingers crossed, they stay healthy and happy. I have three healthy children, a good husband, a nice house and job, but my backpack is full.

Spontaneously, she goes on about the 'super bond' she has with her mother. Mother used to be 'wise' and a pleaser. Her parents divorced when she was 15. Mother has since become weak and sad. Iris has always tried to cheer her up by caring for her emotionally, as Mum had ended several relationships. She finds her mother a bit naive and childish. 'Always that heartbreak!' Mother used to be her God, however.

In her own words:

After my parents' divorce, I suffered immensely. I had narcolepsy. It turned out to be stress. I am the elder of two. With my younger brother, I have a strong bond. He attempted suicide with pills when he was sixteen. Afterwards, we grew more vital towards each other. He is gay. My father is a womaniser. He has always had mistresses. He took me to his dates as an alibi. I had to wait in the bathroom while he did his thing. I told Mum that at the time. Followed an on/off period between them. They separated because of me, but I also brought them together each time. Around that time, I had a boyfriend, Bert. Mother allowed me to do a lot, including, for instance, staying over at his place. The father of that boyfriend was Roger. I thought he was a sweet man. I also thought he was a good partner for my mother. One day, that man started kissing me. I didn't stop that. He looked like my father. In retrospect, Roger had two faces. He was a successful businessman but also an alcoholic and whoremonger. Three months later, he killed himself. I slept with my mother for a long time then; I was afraid Roger was still alive.

As a child, she was precocious and always the smartest in the class. During puberty, she did everything that was not allowed: crawling out the window and going out, smoking joints daily. Her school results slipped, and she dropped from classical humanities to technical education. The mother is an office worker. Iris describes her as a very gentle, warm, and emotional woman. She is said to be 'a bit manic depressive' and consulted with several psychiatrists and fortune-tellers. According to Iris, she put her children first, which made her father feel inadequate and seek attention from other women. 'Mother is not much for sex.'

Father is a professional soldier. She can be herself much more easily with him. She can speak her mind to him entirely; he can stand anything. She calls him a 'handy Harry' and a man for all seasons. After Bert, Fleur fell 'madly in love' with Erik, a man seven years her senior. She moved in with him at 17. She felt big and robust; on top of that, she kept his household running. He often cheated on her, but she could tolerate everything from him. 'He determined everything.'

Finally, however, she began to feel increasingly like his 'hostage'. She then moved out independently and behaved differently towards men: more articulate and on an equal footing. She has been married for several years to a man who has his own business. She calls him quiet and gentle but also ambitious and career-oriented. He is the antithesis of Erik. They have three children. Sexually, the relationship is at a low ebb. 'I want to', but neither takes much initiative. 'The flame has been out for a long time.' And, 'In all my roles, I still feel best as a mother'.

Iris came to me weekly for face-to-face psychoanalytic therapy for about three years. She always talked incessantly, was always cheerful, and tried to be a pleasant and entertaining patient. She was sensitive to the slightest sign of diminished attention or interest on my part and regularly expressed concern about my fatigue, perceived or otherwise. This was seen in connection with her relationship with her mother, from whom she was simultaneously becoming increasingly detached.

Throughout therapy, various negative feelings towards the mother came up. The first were related to parentification. Iris felt that the roles had been reversed emotionally. She had to take care of her mother emotionally more than vice versa. Then again, negative feelings related to the mother's self-centredness. Many examples were given where the mother was more concerned with her feelings than Iris's. There was definitely a lot of Oedipal rivalry, too. In the end, after all, Iris loved her father. He was a solid, independent figure who took charge of their outings. They went on exciting adventures, but Iris always anxiously kept her pleasant experiences hidden from her mother. Her father fixation also became clear along the way. She fell for older and/or dominating men and she did everything in her power to be desired by them as a prima donna and to be carried in their hands as a First Lady. However, the proverbial bumps and bruises started to weigh more with time.

With her husband as a 'reasonable' choice, she put the passionate and turbulent woman in her on hold. For many years, she focused excessively on caring for her husband and children. Also, in a clash, she supported Mum or jumped to spare her even the least hurt.

When the underlying motives were sufficiently exposed, she met an attractive and decent colleague at work for whom she left her husband. The couple parted on a quiet and amicable note, and a few consultations after the discontinued psychotherapy indicated that her current relationship is a hit on all counts. She says this with her eyebrows raised meaningfully.

### Greta—Feeling Instead of Turmoil

A 30-year-old woman who used to pursue art education but has been working in counselling for many years (to her great satisfaction) falls flat:

I was hospitalised because of the problems with my ex-boyfriend. I was there for three years. He terrorised me, beat me, stomped me, controlled me. However, I can't let go of him very well. Still, not completely. It can't go on like this.

Previously, from adolescence, she had been in a steady relationship with a 'good' boy with whom she got on well but with whom she constantly had to 'pull the cart' herself. 'I had to wear the trousers. I was his mother.'

She did not see much good in her new partner right away, but they clicked when they chatted, and she found him to be 'someone exciting'. This was partly owing to his artistic appearance and activities. They had many adventures together and made grand plans, but nothing came of a joint venture. Over time, her life revolved around this boyfriend; now that she has tried to break up with him, her world is empty.

Greta is the second of three children. Things never went well between her parents. 'Father was short-tempered, and mother drew blood from under his nails and played the victim.' They divorced when Greta was an adolescent, and her mother has a new partner with whom Greta says she has a good relationship. Mother is described as an overprotective type. She is full of good intentions and a sponge for other people's problems, but she cannot listen well and gets upset, hurt, or shocked by the slightest thing. Greta has always idealised her mother as if she were perfect. Lately, however, Mother has fallen off her pedestal somewhat.

Father has worked his way up to a position of responsibility. He is wiser and more calculated than her mother but struggles with bipolar disorder, for which he is in psychiatric treatment. 'We experienced very turbulent times with him.'

As early as in her preschool years, Greta did not feel good. She did not like going to preschool. There was little warmth there, and the rules were too strict. She was fearful of failure. In primary school, she fared better. 'There was more of a care factor there; I always needed much attention.' From secondary school onwards, she was very insecure. Moreover, during puberty, she took a wrong path, running away from school and home, using drugs, and sleeping with all kinds of friends and girlfriends. She felt misunderstood and abandoned until she found more of a footing with her first (as said, 'good') sweetheart. She feels she has always had to care for her mother, father, and sweetheart. 'I feel guilty when I do something for myself!'

By our standards, Greta was in inpatient psychotherapy for an extremely short time, barely two months. The treatment environment aims to provide a sufficiently safe, stable, and predictable maternal environment so that many patients can ground themselves there. They need to feel sufficiently at home to expose themselves, shed their cloaks of habitual defence mechanisms, and see the feelings and sensitivities stemming from their life history (including early childhood).

Greta, however, hardly bonded, was very volatile, and was often unjustifiably absent. At weekends, there was a constant off-and-on situation with her boyfriend. Her mind told her to leave him, but he exerted an almost fatal attraction on her.

It is hard for others to believe, but anyone born in Siberia gets homesick for Siberia. Greta had grown up with a hyperemotional and, therefore, overexcited mother who (though very caring) was not responsive to her inner needs. 'When I wept, my mother wept with me.' Father was sometimes very temperamental and overactive, and the relationship between the parents was very turbulent. Greta would have benefited from more peace and stability but, on the other hand, is addicted to toxic stimuli and/or excitation, as it were. No doubt, the famous Lacanian *jouissance* is at play here: a combination of suffering and pleasure underlying repetition compulsion. In my *The Spirit of the Drive*, I described its neuropsychoanalysis.

On the other hand, the factor of parentification is also at play. From an early age, Greta felt called to relieve the emotional needs of others, not least her parents. She has limited reflective and mentalising ability and a habitual tendency to action. She did not return after a weekend, and, apart from a crisis phone call to the night shift a few months later, we heard nothing more from her.

## Henri—a Time Bomb

> I became depressed ten years ago at the transition from high school to university. It all happened abruptly. I had few friends. I went to the GP and to a psychologist each time and was given medication and psychotherapy. It's always the same pattern. I feel a disconnection with reality. This doesn't go away. I live in a dream world. It all doesn't seem real. I don't feel connected to people. This also tricks me in work situations. I keep getting fired. I have lost my personality, am very insecure, feel attacked and cannot defend myself. I am the dupe, but I must kick it off anyway.

This 30-something with rather an adolescent appearance currently works in the hospitality industry. He tried several university courses and did some work here and there, but never for more than a year. He has been living with his parents again for about two years. They are said to be very protective and find it hard to let him go. 'I blame them, but I can't blame them.' They are both very loving but suffocating figures. 'I am the product of shy people.'

Henri is the youngest of three and somewhat the afterthought. Father is an engineer. He is described as a lovely, gentle, aloof man from a farming background. He can also be harsh. 'He "forgets" my problems and background. He has trouble understanding me.' Mother is a housewife and is described as a lovely woman. She is the driving force of the house. She is said to be quite dominant, though. 'My problem is her problem. When I have difficulties, she is also in it, so I keep everything to myself and bottle it up.'

Henri had been in a relationship with Ilse, two years older, for two years. The initiative came from her; he felt somewhat pressured. He also found her 'a bit radical'. He also had a relationship with a girl five years younger for over a year. She said crude things about his parents. For instance, she insinuated that Henri had something sexual with his mother...

In his history, he mentions that he never quarrelled with his parents. From kindergarten, he kept himself apart. He did not mix with the group. 'I didn't join the dance.' He had a single friend with whom he got on well during primary school. It all went pretty okay. From secondary school onwards, he felt less comfortable and suffered from dormant depression. He calls it 'nostalgia, melancholy'. He always felt very lonely, had a small group of friends, and felt lost and abandoned on losing this connection when he transitioned to higher education. He finds university 'a mass affair' and has difficulty socialising there. It's all college graduates. They see him as a weirdo. 'It never clicks.' He wants to be hospitalised but cannot do this to his parents. They would not understand. They forget how serious his problems are. He tries not to think about it. 'I can't think, or I'll lose myself. I get super crazy.' He also has compulsive thoughts. For instance, he thinks it is his fault that people in Africa are starving. He seems to have to bear all the suffering of the world. In contact, Henri makes an avoidant, even schizoid, impression. Impassive on the surface, a tremendous aggressive charge is palpable in him. He seems armed to the teeth. A smile is impossible. Grimness prevails, but he seems to suffer from these negative feelings. Everyone seems distant. Presumably, he is keeping them safe from his own destructive, if not murderous, impulses. He comes to consult only three times.

I suggest an inpatient psychotherapy admission for him after the second interview. This way, he would be away from his parents, which should allow him to better reflect on his relationship with them. It would also help to restructure his very avoidant attachment. He sounds desperate and, when asked, he does appear to have very concrete suicide plans. Working out these deep-seated personality problems reveals itself to be long-term work. Impulsive breakthroughs are also to be feared. Henri agrees with this proposal and says he can empathise with such arguments. Yet he cannot or dare not take the step, to spare his parents. 'I don't want them to feel bad or guilty about their son being hospitalised to psychiatry.'

The fact that his aggression (or even hate) causes Henri to keep others at a safe enough distance seems obvious. Still, when translating and editing this portrait so many years later, I wonder if an element of autism spectrum diagnosis was overlooked. Knowledge and recognition of this (aspect of) psychopathology have increased significantly. Contrary to all psychoanalytic theories about childhood autism, I have come to regard it as a neurocognitive developmental disorder—a (Lacanian) 'real' element disturbing and undermining symbolic-imaginary processing. It is like a grain of sand that needs to be found to mitigate its invisible yet troublesome impact on a psychosocial life that constantly fails to run smoothly. It can lead to 'real' exhaustion and exasperation.

## Jimmy—the Tough Guy

Jimmy is an 18-year-old who was referred by his former youth psychiatrist for drug use, anger outbursts, depressive tendencies, and post-traumatic symptoms. He is the eldest in a three-person family, with a half-brother and a half-sister. His mother is a housewife. She has been in many relationships, and so Jimmy has had as many as 'six fathers'. He speaks of them with a mixture of abandonment, resentment, and rebellion.

His natural father left his mother during her pregnancy. With her, there is a somewhat insecure bond. Sometimes, he clings to her; other times, he takes a tough, pseudo-independent macho stance as a partner and protector. He was a busy and hyperactive child, aggressively ill-treated and sexually abused by one of his stepfathers. From puberty, he developed a drug habit, hung out with gangs, and showed wanton and oppositional behaviour, to be understood as a defence against abandonment, anger, and depression, as well as traumatic fears.

He was in treatment for years in fits and starts, sometimes (semi)residential, sometimes as an outpatient. He experienced remarkable evolution, especially in terms of bonding and trust. He could tell his story and became calmer, more thoughtful, and more nuanced in his dealings with others. Gradually, he dared to feel small and scared now and then, and show it. He did have fleeting promiscuous contacts, where he made a sport of picking up (preferably older) women on the street, conquering them, and then dropping them.

Treatment was derailed as a result of a relapse into taking speed, which resulted in traffic aggression on several occasions. An evil internalised offender object then took hold of him, and he could be very abusive or intimidating towards others.

During this phase, as a therapist, I had a nightmare in which I was locked in a house with a dangerous and violent psychopath. It was an excellent example of what Heinrich Racker calls concordant countertransference. The therapist becomes owned by the patient's feelings and tendencies. By reflecting on these and mentalising them, the therapist can translate them and present them to the patient in a more digestible form. During this period, we were forced to suspend treatment for a while because of a severe incident of aggression. Jimmy may have felt so rejected and abandoned by this that he stopped attending scheduled consultations.

Several years later, I received a letter from the prison asking for admission, which was refused. A few more years later, I saw him several times when he was in his mid-30s. By now, he had established a solid relationship with a slightly older girlfriend with whom he lived. By her account, he took sweet and exemplary care of her children from an earlier relationship. He was a blue-collar worker and could rant furiously in conversations about his boss exploiting the workers. Yet he had worked at the same place for several years and managed (albeit bluntly and swaggeringly) to solve difficulties and denounce abuses.

Women are overrepresented in psychiatry, and men are overrepresented in prison. Technically, women's psychopathology is called autoplastic, and men's is alloplastic. Women literally or figuratively cut into their own flesh; men cut into others'. It ties in with a Lacanian *bon mot*: the woman is the symptom of the man, and the man is havoc for the woman.

Instead of reacting depressively, 'unhappy' boys develop behavioural disorders. Anxious and/or depressive contents are usually hidden behind this totally different and often misunderstood manifestation. Instead of understanding, they tragically collide with (sometimes even legal) condemnation. Within a clinical psychotherapeutic treatment environment, Jimmy settled down somewhat. For the first time in his life, there was development in terms of mental processes and basic safety, which led to a less disjointed and disordered life.

## Gusta—the Importance of Doing Nothing

Gusta is the eldest of five. She has two brothers and two half-brothers. The mother was deprived of parental rights because of emotional and physical abuse and neglect (one of her sons consequently suffered a double skull fracture when he was only 18 months old). The mother was 'never punished' and blamed it on her bad childhood, which the patient does not accept at all.

The father is described as a pedantic tyrant who is emotionally destructive and physically abusive. Gusta is full of anger and hatred towards him. He is currently said to be serving jail time for sexual offences with minors. Her grandparents took Gusta in. She was well cared for by her own account, but her upbringing was rigid, and she was significantly restricted. 'I felt like I was in a golden cage.'

She was incredibly close to her grandfather. He was strict and hot-tempered but could also be sweet. 'I could chat with him and he would reassure me.' By no means did she have the childhood and adolescence of her peers. There are some family psychiatric antecedents in terms of depression and suicide attempts. The whole family is said to be on the hot-tempered and sometimes even violent side.

From childhood, Gusta never felt good; she was constantly bullied everywhere. She would have preferred to be a boy. 'Those are left alone more.' She was married for several years to Gerard, who cheated on her several times. Currently, she is both living alone and single. She works as a home care assistant. She has many physical problems related to Crohn's disease. She has back problems from lifting patients. She is (also) physically wrecked and broken.

She had been in clinical psychotherapy for barely two months. She broadly told her story and integrated very smoothly into the living group, where she told everyone (including in, and especially outside, therapy hours) about the most emotional or intimate problems. She did not get much further than venting or evacuating her negative feelings, only throwing herself somewhat fleetingly into all kinds of activities. She was unable to build a more reflective mode. When she had come sufficiently 'to her senses', she wanted to resume work immediately. 'When I can care for people, I forget about my problems.' She started supportive therapy at the hospital with Monique, a 'nice madame' from a nearby centre for mental healthcare (later: CMHC). A few years later, she crossed the street to come and shake my hand and thank me. 'I no longer run from one doctor to another, and I still go to Monique every fortnight!'

A psychodynamic approach can also be basic. We did little more than let her calm down, pour out her heart, and use the admission as a springboard for out-patient therapy in which non-specific factors such as positive acceptance, warmth, empathy, and a constant and reliable therapeutic relationship played the leading role. In patients with such serious histories, a listening ear does more wonders than all kinds of (even the most drastic) medical interventions. As the 17th-century Jesuit Baltazar Gracián says somewhere in his *Hand Oracle*, you need as much intelligence to do nothing as to do something.

## Nicole—Rolling Stones

This 30-year-old administrative clerk in the army says she has been in the doldrums for years with back and depression symptoms and has already tried all kinds of things. She feels now is the time to grit her teeth and bite the bullet because the pit is getting deeper and deeper, and more needs to be done. She first visited a psychologist when she was 6 and, at 15, she took an overdose of medication, after which she was in PWGH for several weeks. About five years ago, she spent several months in a women's refuge and has been in outpatient therapy ever since.

Nicole is the youngest of four and the only daughter. She and her eldest brother have a good relationship. The other two have almost wholly severed contact with their parents. They all lead very separate lives and rarely see each other except on official occasions. The brother who comes before her has always been her mother's favourite, and Nicole begged her for attention, which she never got. Instead, she feels rejected by her mother. She was implicitly and explicitly told that she was unwanted, the nail in her mother's coffin, and that everything was always her fault. Her mother allegedly once had her by the throat and tried to strangle Nicole. This incident continues to haunt her as if it were yesterday.

Nicole says she has separation anxiety. As a result, she clings to people or, conversely, has a great fear of getting attached to anyone. After secondary school, she took a higher degree in interior decoration and found her niche in it. However, she was allergic to specific products and thus had to give up this rewarding outlet.

Mother is described as a busybody who comments on everything and everyone. She lives on gossip and slander. Everything must always go precisely as she wishes, 'because otherwise there will be trouble'. Father is a civil servant. He is a true cultural man with a big heart for young people. He is famous and liked everywhere because he is a socially minded figure. Yet he was hardly present within the family. All in all, she feels he left her with her mother and that he did not intervene, even though she thought she was in her mother's clutches. She always hoped her parents would divorce, but this never happened.

As a child, Nicole was tremendously lonely. She had few or no friends. She spent a lot of time in her room doing puzzles and reading. At school, she was a difficult pupil. She often got into arguments with her fellows and teachers. She was 'kicked out' of the youth movement and, in terms of performance, she dropped from general secondary to preprofessional school.

From adolescence, there was regular and heavy cannabis use to 'get away'. She had many casual sexual contacts and liked to seduce and feel desired. She was in a relationship with a 20-year-older divorced man and father of three children for about two years. He was an alcoholic, physically and psychologically aggressive, and, above all, extremely jealous and possessive. She lived with him in an atmosphere of constant fear and violence and had to flee to a safe house.

Psychoanalysis has already gone through several paradigmatic switches. Even during Freud's lifetime, there were the affect-trauma model, the topographical model (unconscious, pre-conscious, conscious), and the structural Id–Ego–Superego model. The drive theory runs like a thread through all three. After that, there is Ego psychology, the object-relational perspective, and the (post)Kleinian and intersubjective two-person psychology.

Currently, a body of thought centred around mentalisation is in the foreground, in which neuroscientific findings, infant research, and attachment research are integrated. Psychoanalytic therapy is not in the least about developmental aid, working on mental functions and processes rather than their contents. According to Freud, progress is only half as significant as it initially appears. Instead, each time, it involves a new map to describe the field or a different lens through which we can better understand clinical phenomena.

Nicole was in inpatient psychotherapy for over a year. Within this maternal environment, attempts are made to recalibrate the attachment system. This 'structural' change is inextricably linked to increased resilience and mentalising abilities that, in their interplay, help increase the patient's psychosocial and psychosexual action radius.

As might be expected, building and maintaining a therapeutic alliance with Nicole proved far from easy. First of all, there was severe negative maternal transference towards both various team members and the (mother) institute in general. There were countless unwarranted and unexcused absences or fugues. In addition, she regularly relapsed into cannabis use with all its toxic consequences for her own and others' safety and trust.

Towards the end of her treatment, she also became embroiled in a blinkered relationship with a fellow group member. He wallowed in an artistic haze and, like her, struggled with a mixture of separation and bonding anxiety. He embodied specific components of her father and acted as a *soulmate* or buddy: they were each other's sounding board, understood each other without words, and could revel in a mutual mirroring that benefitted their sense of self (value). We tried to refer one or other partner in the couple elsewhere, but they 'chose' their relationship over therapy. 'Love is the Drug' sings Roxy Music, although Nicole was more of a Rolling Stones fan.

## Catherine—the University of Life

We hospitalised this 35-year-old woman, who is highly skilled and works in the care sector, after she had already 'worn out' about five psychotherapists. She says she has gained insights but, on the other hand, feels she has not yet made any progress. Manifestly, her problems started in adolescence with binge eating and vomiting alternating with anorectic periods. These never significantly impacted her weight and were, therefore, never noticed by the outside world. However, things were closely monitored by the mother.

After three years of courtship, she married a decent and highly educated man at 28. She says he epitomises poise and common sense but also finds him boring and annoying. Consequently, she has cheated on him several times with various lovers.

Catherine is the youngest of five children. Her mother was in education but took early retirement to care for her grandchildren. As such, she is described as very concerned and caring. Catherine has always looked up to her mother very much. Her father is a retired electrician. She and he always had a more distant relationship. He is said to have been absent often because of busy professional activities and is emotionally closed and taciturn.

Catherine never had many boyfriends or girlfriends. 'We are all not very social, except father.' She was very much on her own and felt inferior to her peers. She felt too fat and 'less cool'. She never fitted in well in groups. She was not in the youth movement, but she did take piano lessons at music school. However, she was never really good at this, nor did she like it, but she tried to live up to expectations. On the other hand, she was always an excellent and exemplary student. Her parents adored and idolised her for being top of the class. She was considered the family's prodigy. Not that she could be proud of this. After all, modesty was strongly encouraged within the family.

Catherine experienced hardly any adolescent turmoil . By her admission, she had no desire to pull herself away from home. She nestled into the domestic cocoon and preferred to stay comfortable and protected. During her higher studies, she achieved very good results. In hindsight, however, she considers this 'parrot work', mere reproduction of pre-digested knowledge.

The problems started as soon as she entered real (professional) life. She was highly uncertain and insecure, constantly afraid of 'falling through the cracks'. Given her high scores, an academic career was open to her, but she allowed herself to slip into jobs that became further and further below her (intellectual) level. In diffuse and difficult-to-specify ways, she also felt frustrated and dissatisfied in her current life. After graduating, she also ended up in a black hole. None of it appealed to her, and she wanted something else.

Behind a brave and conformist façade, she hides a would-be femme fatale who feasts on the 'I only have eyes for you, baby' that is the hallmark of infatuations. She clings to the security and protection offered to her by her husband. 'He takes care of me like a chick.' On the other hand, she sneakily tries to have all kinds of wild adventures. She can feel like a prima donna for as long as it lasts and enjoys being treated like a princess.

Catherine had been in clinical psychotherapy for over a year. Because of her frail and adolescent appearance, she had great success with male fellow patients. She had a relationship with one of them. Behind his façade of an oppositional free spirit was a little boy who had always missed his mother's love and appreciation. Together, they went on several clandestine outings the deep narcissistic, rather than erotic, significance of which became increasingly evident in the psychotherapeutic conversations.

With the help of pre-professional training and employment counselling, she started more training during her admission. Following her discharge, she has been in weekly psychotherapy, face-to-face, for about three years. The eating disorders turned out to be the tip of the iceberg of ambivalent feelings towards, and independence struggles with, the mother. Catherine realises she has been hiding behind her books all her life. She has played hooky from the 'university of life' by staying hidden behind her mother's skirts. There are all kinds of psycho-social skills that most children learn in the (literal or figurative) playground which she has hardly developed. Her 'adventures' are a meagre consolation for the frustrations she feels at a childish dependency in which she has felt trapped since her earliest childhood.

It is one thing to see why all grew crooked or inadequate. Her mother's excessive care, her father's absence, and her school results led to her being idolised. In a kind of heliotropism, she grew towards the light and the sun until her head proved too big and her stem and base too narrow, and she toppled over on the threshold of summer. Now, she toils for every inch of ground gained. What we did not learn spontaneously and playfully as children, 365 days a year, is—adult-wise—a chore we must do to catch up with growth. High intelligence aside, it is possible that we will continue to drag a lot of 'backwardness' into adulthood.

## Irene—Experiencing versus Functioning

This coquettish 55-year-old woman was referred for inpatient psychotherapy by a psychiatrist whom she consulted several times. Eight years ago, she experienced a brief admission to a PWGH service following a family crisis and assault at the hands of her then-partner. 'I want to rest, function again, not be in pain, sleep.'

The eldest of four daughters, she threw herself into mothering the two youngest. Father worked his way up to business manager and passed away several years ago. He had tremendous discipline; 'they called him a little Hitler'. He would have preferred sons and showed little affection to his daughters. 'Women are good to sit at a desk.' His will was law, and everyone feared him: he was violent and dealt hard blows. He was a loner from a huge family where everyone had to make it.

The mother is described as calm and indifferent. According to the patient, she is not very sensible; her conversation is limited to chatting over coffee. Superficially, their bond is good, but 'she stood me up'. She also favoured the patient's younger sister, who won several beauty pageants. Compared with her, Irene felt cornered: 'I wasn't allowed to be seen'.

From a young age, she was lonely and took refuge in a fantasy world, drawing and painting. She didn't have many friends, had to help clean and wash at home, and was a scared follower who always let herself be taken advantage of everywhere. After secondary school, she worked as a secretary for several doctors for many years. She ran the practice there, was a maid-of-all-work, and greatly criticised the seriousness of their practice management. 'It was a genuine factory. Patients had to draw numbers there, like at the butcher's.'

In recent years, she has worked in home care. There, she gets the most demanding clients, for whom she puts herself out, while younger colleagues 'do and take it much more at ease'. At the age of 20, she married her first steady sweetheart. He was a self-employed entrepreneur, always out and about. He had several extramarital affairs, and, after his father's death, the business went bankrupt owing to his mismanagement. Their three sons are doing just fine.

A few years before, Irene was divorced by mutual consent. By her own account, she barely resisted and was on the street empty-handed in no time. She allegedly went through postnatal depression after the birth of her youngest son. In the family, there is some occurrence of melancholic and sensitive traits, but, as far as we know, there have been no psychiatric hospitalisations.

All psychology and psychopathology result from a not quite distinguishable intertwining of three dimensions. First is the biological: the genes, the body, and the brain. Unlike many somatic phenomena where biological abnormalities can be made visible or measurable and, thus, act as 'markers' for this or that diagnosis, such evidence for the psychological is lacking.

To evaluate the biological impact, we have to make do with 'circumstantial evidence'—such as, a familial occurrence or specific pathognomonic signs of disease (imperative auditory hallucinations in schizophrenia, disturbances in vital and/or cognitive functions in major mood disorders). Second, there is the imaginary register humans have in common with animals. We can refer to attachment, courtship behaviour, mimicry, or other behaviour by which we try to survive and procreate. Finally, the typical human register is symbolic, with its language based on law and convention. It definitively separates us from a (supposed) immediacy to which we long to return, the *Real Thing* to which now pleasure and sometimes even passion or madness drive us.

Within clinical psychotherapy, these causal factors are weighted so that treatment is based on them judiciously and proportionately. In some patients, biological and/or drug treatment plays a leading role. In most, it plays a valuable and primarily transient, secondary role, keeping the suffering workable and liveable while waiting for the fruits of psychotherapy to be reaped. In reality, in psychiatric suffering, low-hanging fruit is rare.

In almost all patients, there is some attachment work. Inner working models stored in our implicit memory come *live on stage* through enactment. The patient's behaviour and acting out must be translated in an attuned way. They are promoted to symptoms or signifiers that can only be understood in the context of the life history and the here-and-now of the total transference situation. History is continuously being written and rewritten, and specific feelings and sensitivities repeat themselves, the (sometimes early) childhood roots of which must be uncovered.

Therapy for patients such as Irene is usually limited to a patch-up approach. Psychopharmaceuticals are prescribed, and there is a supportive and covert approach seeking a return to work and 'normal' functioning as soon as possible.

In clinical psychotherapy, there is an investment in the inside. How does the patient feel? How do they experience the outside world? Are there things in this that are repetitive and from which they suffer? The intention is to allow the inner world to unfold and to try to understand, with united effort, how much the past and history leave their mark. Giving them 'a place' creates the distance necessary to free themself from hitherto ill-fated patterns. The stereotypical is replaced by stereovision.

Irene became aware of the lack of attention, understanding, and love she experienced because of her mother. She was 'programmed' to obey a *Führer* and constantly found herself in a parentified position where she had to go out of her way to care for others while being left out in the cold with her own needs. She tried to adjust where necessary as she gained insight into these stumbling blocks.

Let's compare life to a road, with turns and intersections, inclines and declines, asphalt and cobblestones, and other road users who are safe or dangerous. Where did I get lost? How did I end up in a cul-de-sac, in the middle of nowhere, or back at the point I left? Driving more to the left or the right makes you arrive, many kilometres on, in a completely different territory to usual.

## Shirley—from Glum to Glam

This 30-year-old woman came for outpatient psychotherapy with a problem of hair loss. Physically, everything had been examined, and no objectifiable abnormalities were found. 'It seems to be caused by stress.' She has been suffering from panic attacks for about five years and was in behavioural therapy treatment with a psychologist for this, while her GP prescribed her several antidepressants. 'I am a real control freak and also very perfectionist. Everything has to be done my way.'

She has been unemployed since the beginning of the year and feels unemployable. 'I would feel trapped.' She received a higher education in the arts and has been with a man her age who has freelanced in show business for four years. The relationship goes 'with ups and downs'. He is absent and out a lot. He comes home at night and sometimes sleeps elsewhere. She often feels lonely and abandoned. When they see each other, they can barely speak to each other. She misses the boys with whom she was on the same wavelength, 'with egos clashing, struggles, inspirations, challenges'. In that sense, she thinks back to her college days with nostalgia. It was an exciting period.

Shirley is an only child. Her mother wanted another child, but, for her father, one was already 'more than enough'. She says her parents do not form a 'typical couple'. Father works in the media. He is not a 'standard dad' but rather a kind of friend. She owes her artistic interests and sensitivity to him. He taught her everything and was her 'big hero' for a long time. She never received punishments or boundaries from him, though.

> With my mother, I have always had a dual relationship. She is irritable, you can't talk to her, you can't be yourself. She has hardly any sense of humour and sees everything in black and white. Contact with her is strained.

Shirley thinks she resembles her father in character. 'Mother recognises father in me.' The parents are divorced. Mother did set boundaries and rules. As a small child, Shirley gravitated more towards her mother. Conversely, the mother echoed her and portrayed her father as a 'bad guy'. She often hoped her parents would divorce, as there were many arguments. Still, she feels she had a happy childhood. She felt good about herself, was sociable, achieved fine school results, and enjoyed popularity.

During adolescence, Shirley resented her mother, who felt she conspired with her father. Shirley obtained a classical humanities degree, and her mother hoped she would become a lawyer. After all, this was her frustrated desire. Shirley pushed through her will and now sometimes feels she has to pay for it in the form of unemployment and financial problems. There is something glum and joyless about her appearance.

According to Robert Hinshelwood, 'Psychiatric institutions exist for people who cannot contain themselves'. They can no longer hide their problems. Not from others and no longer from themselves either. The issues (and their causes) are sometimes laid on thickly. How different it is with many patients who come to consult in an outpatient setting. At first glance, it is not immediately clear what exactly is wrong. There are various complaints or symptoms, but what do they mean?

Shirley came weekly for about three years. Some themes came alternately to the fore throughout her psychotherapy, and their interrelationships would gradually appear. Most important was undoubtedly the problematic relationship with her mother. In her story, she was sometimes super sweet and supportive, at other times very cool and dismissive. Shirley was rarely, if ever, allowed to experience genuine empathy. With her school achievements, she was sometimes her mother's showcase; then again, she felt envy and jealousy emanating from her mother because of her success or ability.

Owing to the poor marital relationship, Shirley was sometimes the head of the household for the mother. Also, her mother could not stomach that things were often very close between father and daughter. On the other hand, the father was phallically weak. In her story, he was instead a lousy boy who played as a musician in all sorts of more or less obscure bands. He was, therefore, *on the road* and had a companionate rather than paternal relationship with his daughter. There was little of 'protect and provide' (as indicators of male maturity).

Her relationship was also discussed at length. It gradually became clear to her that her partner showed some traits of both mother and father. They had the same musical tastes, but he was unpredictable and changeable, leading a bohemian existence with a lot of artistic verve that offered her little security or grip. In the middle phase of her therapy, she summed things up as follows: 'I have a mother who is not a mother, a father who is not a father and a partner who is not a partner.'

A critical Eureka moment was the following seemingly trivial incident. After not seeing her for several months, Shirley ran into her mother on the street. At least she *thought* she saw her mother, because she was not sure. 'How is it possible that I don't even know if she is my mother or not!' The alienation and *Unheimlich* feeling that resulted from this doubt occupied her for several consecutive sessions, during which countless moments of empathic failure or a 'bad connection' with her mother were reviewed.

In the course of her psychotherapy, Shirley detached herself from both parents. She looked for and found a 'right distance' that best reflected psychological and emotional realities. She also broke off the relationship with her partner. She greatly feared working somewhere full-time and 'permanently' for a long time. She was afraid of getting stuck (again) in a tricky situation.

How many times had she longed for her parents to divorce—in her view, the only way out of a painful and unsolvable impasse?

In the last year, she found steady work in the creative sector and purposefully built a circle of friends. Towards the end, her somewhat dishevelled looks had given way to a sexy woman who had grown considerably, not only through but also on top of her ever-higher heels.

## Sharon—a Nose with Teeth

Sharon has been briefly hospitalised at a PWGH service many times because of depression and suicidality. She quickly recovered thanks to a whole arsenal of antidepressants but relapsed into the same symptoms every time. She was, therefore, referred for—as it is called there—'long-term' treatment.

She is the second in a family of three. Both her brothers do just fine. The father is a municipal worker. She has a good relationship with him. She can count on him. He is also understanding. Her mother is a blue-collar worker. With her, the contact/connection is a lot less promising. She is of Polish origin, and they don't understand each other very well. Mother would 'nag and complain' a lot. During her primary school days, a dog bit Sharon in the face. Around the age of 12, Sharon already felt depressed and thought of suicide. There were many arguments with the mother. At school, everything was going well. She studied admin and sales. She has always had somewhat low self-esteem. 'I don't like (to see) myself.' She constantly felt like she was failing, falling short.

She had several relationships. First, there was Geoffrey, between the ages of 15 and 20. He was violent and gave Sharon a bloody nose on several occasions. She dropped all her friends for him, and, finally, he left and cheated on her. There followed Kevin, who went through manic periods and needed psychiatric admission. She lived with him for about three years, and he abandoned her for another woman. Finally, there was Bick, with whom she ran a neighbourhood supermarket and who left her for a much older Thai woman. She felt hurt by all this (as a woman). To make matters worse, she had a traffic accident that caused aesthetic damage to her face. Her nose was deformed beyond recognition as a result, in her opinion. With regard to her self-image, this was the proverbial straw that broke the camel's back. She has been working as a salaried cleaning lady for the last year. Before that, she was a shop assistant at various places. She has been single for two years.

In long-lasting alternating depressive symptoms described under the heading of dysthymic disorder, three significant types occur. There is neurotic depression, where inner conflicts stealthily claim a lot of energy, where aggression is directed at the self, or where the Superego imposes a specific penalty on the person concerned. There is abandonment depression, where early childhood deficits begin to take their revenge sooner or later. However, there are also narcissistic problems where there are disturbances in the regulation of self-esteem, self-worth, self-image, or self-love.

We live in a time when psychiatric journals and associations talk about biological treatment methods, neuroscientific explanations, or high-tech neurostimulation where one acts linearly on the 'guilty' regions of the brain. In a way, all this defies imagination. After all, you don't have to be a genius to understand that all these interventions don't change one iota about conscious or unconscious psychogenic causality as it plays out in dysthymic disorders.

It is sometimes said that it is not which drugs are prescribed but *who* prescribes them that explains their effect (including the placebo effect). The quality of the therapeutic relationship makes a great difference indeed and, as a non-specific or generic factor, plays a crucial role in any counselling.

In reality, Sharon lacked adequate mirroring because of her mother. This plays a role in building basic safety and mentalising ability and setting up a stable and positive self-image. Sharon was hurt or maimed. The fact that she was repeatedly unhappy with her choice of partner appeared to have everything to do with her extremely low self-esteem. If a man paid any attention to her, she at once clung to him and allowed herself to be slavishly, even (seemingly) masochistically, mistreated for far too long.

She was in clinical psychotherapy with us for barely three months. It was sufficient to distil the sensitivities described from her life history and work with them within an empathic and supportive therapy.

Because of her limited financial resources, we directed her to a local CMHC for further outpatient therapy. There, she was supervised weekly by a caring social worker while she came to me infrequently for psychiatric and psychoanalytic process counselling. Two years later, she is medication-free. She is online dating, calmly. When men take a somewhat overly forward or brash attitude towards her, she knows how to put them in their place. For instance, she said with a cheeky smile: 'If they act harassingly, I'll bite their nose off'.

## Dirk—God Is a DJ

A boyish 40-something comes for outpatient consultations because he has been uncomfortable for several months. 'I am married with four children and in love with someone else. Things are also going badly at work.' In recent years, he has started playing tennis. Caroline, the woman who runs the tennis club's cafeteria, is a 'cool madam', and he fantasises about her. One of the other tennis players is also in love with her, and that man is 'likewise'(!) divorced. He is jealous of it. He also feels guilty towards his wife. He finds warmth and security with her. 'She is a good mother.' She is a lovely woman with a great sense of humour. He has also previously fallen in love with another woman who travelled alone. 'I fall in love with strong, independent women. Women with balls.'

Dirk is the youngest of four children and the only son. His mother was already in her 40s when he was born. His father was a grocer. He was a charming, well-liked figure who loved parties and had a lot of fun. He died when Dirk was 12. 'There were more than 2,000 people at his funeral.' His father did think he was a 'spoilt shit'. Indeed, Dirk was indulged and spoilt by his mother and older sisters. He remembers being in love in kindergarten. He played the tough one to seduce the girls. 'Teasing girls is asking for love.'

He was always effortlessly among the top pupils in the class in primary school. In secondary school, he was the cock of the walk. He had a big mouth but surrounded himself with, and stood behind, tough guys and rebellious types. 'I needed a lot of attention. I showed off everywhere.' As long as his father was alive, there was plenty. Afterwards, however, substantial financial problems arose. His mother was sad and wallowed in self-pity, and Dirk had to assist her.

In adolescence, Dirk started working in the catering industry. This gave him plenty of pocket money and allowed him to 'play the big guy'. He fondly recalls his heyday behind the turntable: 'God is a DJ!' He tried higher education, but, because he was earning so much money, he neglected his studies. He was hostile to authority. By his own admission, he had terrible manners and laughed in teachers' faces.

He has built a supply company for the hospitality industry with two partners. Dirk mainly takes care of promotion and contacts, as business is not his strongest point in the narrower sense. Fortunately, he can count on the others for this. 'They are men I can lean on.' In that context, he unsolicitedly mentions: 'I am looking for a father figure'. He feels unbalanced, especially since the mother's death a few years earlier. He feels restless and dissatisfied. While he drinks habitually, his alcohol consumption is running out of control. He likes to be in a stupor because he feels a bit 'high'.

All in all, Dirk was in weekly face-to-face psychotherapy for about two years. For a lot of the time, he was very playful and charming in the conversations. In several sessions, I experienced him as a stand-up comedian who performed a one-man show with the necessary irony and self-mockery. He often made me laugh, but I tried to keep my reflective attitude. He was a comical little fellow who elicited tender, affectionate feelings.

It became clear that he had been the centre of female attention for many years. He had received an overdose of love and attention to which he had, in a way, become addicted. In his eyes, his father was a kind of famous celebrity whose star had been extinguished on the threshold of Dirk's adolescence. He had hardly interfered in Dirk's upbringing, so Dirk experienced little or no authority or boundaries. In his adolescence, Dirk took on his father's mantle. He always put his money where his mouth was, but, when it came down to it, he felt insecure and small and had trouble 'standing his ground' when faced with difficulties or conflicts. He needed drink to find his courage or try to ditch other men.

On the one hand, he needed a kind of mother, a wife by the fireplace, a role his spouse fulfilled. But one woman was not enough for him. Was he not used to being loved, beloved, and adored by several women? He gradually discovered that he was particularly attracted to women who seemed sexually adventurous and who dared to go out into the world and battle like Amazons.

It was quite a revelation to him when he found out that, despite their female anatomy, they were *father figures* who kept him at bay and from whom he could derive phallic powers. Analysing his fantasies concerning Caroline broke the spell. Professionally, he downsized to take more care of his wife and children. When his wife developed health problems, he took over the torch in terms of housekeeping and raising the kids and, in taking on care and responsibility, he discovered a whole new kind of satisfaction. 'I have never felt so much like a man before.'

## Alexander—Blablabla or Bangbangbang?

Alexander was hospitalised in crisis following an impending relationship break-up. From the time of his telephone application, he had announced himself as a sex addict. He is 30, but still very boyish in appearance. He begins his story as follows:

> Ten years ago, I went to a prostitute. It left me with an addiction. Two months later, I returned. That's how I ended up in a vicious cycle. I finally told my girlfriend. Then, I was able to stop for a year. Now it's back there. Sandra thinks I should work on it more thoroughly now.

Alexander is the youngest of three. He has two sisters, who are seven and four years older than him. He says he comes from a good family. He has always received a lot of warmth, love, and attention. 'Maybe even too much.' Even unsolicited, his mother tries to predict all his needs and wishes. He describes her as a somewhat busy and very emotional woman who cannot let go. He describes his father as a rational person. He only makes small talk and mostly keeps a low profile. It isn't easy to talk to him about his feelings. All in all, he is somewhat aloof and reserved.

Asked about his problems, Alexander finds that he is somewhat stuck with his mother. He remembers perfectly well his first day of school. He was scared of the new environment and cried all day. During his preschool and primary school years, he was looked after at noon and after school by a lovely, friendly nanny, whom he invariably calls his 'foster mother'. Only from secondary school onwards did he have to be independent. By this, he meant eating at school, taking the bus alone, and so on. He did not like going to school and he did not like studying. He felt more serious and mature than his peers. He drew a lot. So, he earned a higher degree in plastic arts and worked as a teacher for several years. He has been living with his girlfriend, Sandra, for several years.

He lets his sexual story begin with the adolescent daughter of the nanny. He fell in love with her during the first years of primary school without daring to speak to anyone about it. All the while, he indulged in erotic and romantic fantasies. 'I was fixated on her.' He attended a boys' school for the first three years of his secondary school education. By his own admission, he was very awkward with girls, afraid of not being accepted. 'I was introverted and reserved.'

During this period, he was constantly on the internet, a euphemism he used for his pornographic interest. 'Other things suffered. I put a lot of time and energy into it at their expense. This was all done in secret.' Also, during this period, he developed a keen interest in the brothels in the neighbourhood. They exerted a 'magnetic' attraction on him. He often cycled past them and excitedly peered at the red-lighted windows.

Alexander was very anxious and nervous during those years. He went to see a psychologist several times, who encouraged him to take real action. He became more open and met his first sweetheart. 'She was everything to me.' She 'played' with his feelings for several months because she was not serious about the relationship. For instance, she also had sexual contact with other boys. In the end, she left him. He then met his current partner. 'She cared about me very much.' Still, during that period, he drank a lot and, under the influence of alcohol, he let a friend persuade him to visit a prostitute. 'It's a mystery how that could have happened. I was traumatised by it.'

Tormented by guilt, he confessed everything to Sandra, and, although she was hurt, she responded surprisingly understandingly. A while later, a slightly older student had feelings for him. He ended up sleeping with her. 'I could hardly say no.' He panicked and at once called his mother and sisters. It dragged on for a while. 'I found it very difficult to let go of that woman,' he said.

In recent years, he has been going to the red-light district almost every day, after work. He walks around looking for new faces. By his admission, he looks for temptation there to be able to resist it. Sometimes, he goes in. Rarely, if ever, does it come to actual sexual contact. He often settles for a striptease. On several occasions, he has gone in, chatted a little, paid, and left.

On the internet, he surfs pornography sites. He is looking for a woman who appeals to him. He does not care about extreme states. It is mainly the excitement of women that turns him on. He doubts his feelings for his girlfriend. However, he always gives plenty of reasons why she is a good match for him. Her maternal qualities (solidity, reliability, security, affection) prevail. He does think she does not take enough initiative sexually. She seems to find sex a lot less important than he does and hardly enjoys it. Or is that his fault and punishment? After all, hasn't he hurt and betrayed her love and trust? For the first few years of their relationship, sexually, 'everything was as it should be'. Nevertheless, he also looked for the sexual elsewhere. So it's not that something is wrong with their relationship.

Alexander was only in inpatient psychotherapy for a few weeks. Enough to calm down, let the crisis at home cool down, and talk a bit about his difficulties. Afterwards, he came to weekly psychotherapy for about five years.

Many different factors related to his problems were discussed. As always, his problem is overdetermined and has multiple causes.

First, there is the close relationship with his mother. She was and is present rather too much. He tries to set a boundary and distance himself from her, with varying degrees of success, although he still needs a mother at the same time. Alexander was somewhat spoilt and overstimulated by her. Two older sisters also treated him maternally. A striking element in his history is that he bathed with the youngest of his older sisters until her adolescence. He secretly admired her full glory and was immersed in warm wetness with her. He can well remember how he hid incipient erections from her or tried to nip them in the bud.

On closer inspection, he could only understand the fact that his parents allowed these intimacies because they repressed or denied the importance of (his) sexuality. At home, sex was a taboo subject. It was not discussed, and he noted that not *Playboy* but the parish magazine adorned the coffee table. He saw his father as a firm and rational but otherwise rather flabby and phallically weak figure. How sharply he contrasted with an uncle who owned a garage where, with the permission and knowledge of his wife, Pirelli calendars full of female beauty adorned the walls!

Alexander gradually became aware of his overly well-behaved and respectful attitude towards girls/women. Unlike many fellow students who went full steam ahead with their artistic careers, he insisted on safety and protection. Sex was something to be kept behind screens (including computer screens), or something about which clear agreements could be reached and for which he had to (or wanted to) *pay* to erase all guilt as much as possible.

Habitually, there was remarkable sexual and aggressive inhibition. Paradoxically, only 'red-light' districts excited him. Indeed, he was usually 'the good' Alexander, who always avoided conflict everywhere and hardly dared to push for his own way.

While sex was initially hardly discussable, even within his relationship, he tried to discuss his desires and fantasies there more. His compulsive brothel visits ebbed away. Only occasionally did he drive past 'to *soak up* the atmosphere'. This was mainly about the perfume of the forbidden and the affirmation of the masculinity he seemed to experience there. While he kept the door/heart open for a different and better woman for a long time, he could engage more fully.

Soon, he will become a father for the second time. With regard to his children's upbringing, he has resolved to talk about sex as much as necessary so that they can give it its proper place, better than before. Only then, he believes, will there be a real sexual revolution!

### Chris—Cape of Good Hope

In his early 20s, this young adult man was hospitalised in a borderline-psychotic and disinhibited, agitated state. His thinking is highly associative, and he cannot stay seated during the introductory interview. His opening line: 'An accumulation of factors has crumpled me'. With regard to higher education, he has done a bit of everything: mechanics, car mechanics, computer science, and industrial sciences. Eventually, he wants to become an engineer, but now he has a 'blackout'. 'Everything is stuck.' He says he sees things that are not there, 'exactly like in a dream'.

Chris is the youngest of three. His mother is in education. He describes her as impulsive and thoughtless. She would pamper him. However: 'I don't want her to clean my pooch'. His father is a technical draughtsman. He is said to be calmer and more thoughtful. 'He is the opposite of mother.' He gives Chris freedom and encourages him but does not impose himself, while his mother drops in on Chris uninvited, (literally) through the back door. He would have experienced both too much and too little love. Too much mothering and too little fathering.

Chris was also the darling of his paternal grandparents. They pampered him, worshipped him. His grandfather, in particular, emerges from his story as a mythical and creative figure. In reality, he recycled textiles, but, in Chris's eyes, he was *larger than life* and produced a powerful impression. With the sister closest to him, there was a very intense and passionate love/hate relationship. They slept in the same room for a long time and they played sexual games that excited him a lot. The father constantly tried to intervene, but, for Chris, it was a game of cat and mouse with him. In retrospect, he feels like his sister's toy and sex object, and, from puberty onwards, she was very dismissive and castrating towards him. He could not resist her verbal and intellectual supremacy at all. He lacked support from a father to pull himself together sufficiently.

From puberty onwards, he appeared as a macho 'bad boy'. He constantly rebelled against teachers with great swagger. He was expelled from school several times. On the other hand, he describes himself as very housebound, but, lately, he feels displaced and uprooted. He has never been in a steady relationship. He considers himself too monomaniacal for that. He does, however, have promiscuous sexual contact. He wants to become an inventor or an artist. Auguste Rodin, for instance, is his idol and role model. Above all, he wants to exhibit. Among other things, he shows me a giant spanner on a large canvas and a wall-wide collage with, as it were, a collection of women in lingerie.

Chris is now a young 40-something. Different phases can be distinguished in his therapeutic process. First, he was in inpatient psychotherapy for about a year. During this first phase, there was a lot of anger and rebellion towards the father and the law. He felt inadequately supported and appreciated by me as a ward psychiatrist; on the other hand, he had sexual contact with several female patients on the ward. To cap it all, he started an affair with a cousin who was temporarily working in our hospital, knowing full well that this was not only figuratively but also literally an incestuous action. Of course, all this was interpreted in an Oedipal context as 'fuck you' behaviour: rebellion against and rivalry with the father, erotic fixation on the mother and sister.

After admission, he underwent three years of outpatient group psychotherapy. He completed a master's degree in engineering, moved into his grandfather's former home, and had several relationships with women, each of which somehow left him hungry. It was never the True One.

He then stayed away for several years and reported back following a telling parapraxis. Meanwhile, at work, he had inserted a glowing rod into a test tube and suffered a severe burn on his hand in the resulting explosion. The sexual and incestuous symbolism was obvious even to himself. He was aware of the danger. However, he had quasi-deliberately sought this 'accident' himself. He had played with fire and had to be punished for this. The decision was made for him. Further analytical work needed to be done.

There followed several years during which he came to me for individual face-to-face psychotherapy every week. Different themes often arose over weeks or months. First came the theme of the prodigy he was to the grandparents. They loved and adored him and were enamoured with his playfulness and creativity. He had felt like a god in the depths of their minds.

There was in him a hard and persistent core of *would-be* Creator. He tried to make something beautiful in various work situations, even when it was not (really) relevant. He wanted to show something (phallic) and gain admiration for it. He clashed with bosses who neither supported nor understood this endeavour—'fat capitalists' (the reader may guess what I look like) for whom everything is only about money.

The desire regularly arose to retreat far from the Western world as a kind of hermit, where he would live off the heavenly dew, so to speak, and indulge in play and creativity. His grandfather was the almighty god-the-father. If you are his son, you share in his divinity. What happens when he dies? *Le roi/Dieu est mort, vive le roi/Dieu!* The king/God is dead; long live the king/God!

Several artists/idols took over the grandfather's position later in life. Time and again, Chris clashed with reality: both in his partner relationships and at work, he had to slow down in terms of omnipotence and posturing. There was a lot of pent-up anger around this, with the lid occasionally flying off the pot, resulting in unreasonable scalding and scenes. There were frustrations and hurt feelings throughout his life and therapy, and, by empathically mirroring them, I could help him digest them. In this way, a grandiose self gradually became increasingly tamed and tempered.

Another theme was the boundless (love of the) mother. Even when he behaved like a tyrant or a terrorist, she continued to love him unconditionally and embrace him lovingly. No matter how 'ugly' he was to her, she always came back. He almost had to turn into a monster to break away from her because, however hard he pecked, he could not break the eggshell in which she continued to cherish him.

Chris has long been afraid of committing to a woman. He feared (as with his mother) becoming her 'little Chris', falling into her power (as with his sister), or missing out on the chance of other and better women. For many years, he had a steady relationship with a kindergarten teacher he eventually married. He enjoyed and benefited, as it were, from the way she treated her infant son from an earlier relationship. On the one hand, she was very caring, loving, and warm. On the other hand, she consistently set clear rules and boundaries. Between them, they now had two children. Initially, he tended to be more of a playmate than a father figure for them. However, he, usually willingly, allowed himself to be corrected and instructed by his wife.

In his mind, he understands the pitfalls and where they come from, but only arduously does he manage to free himself from his childish reactions and needs. Time and again, he contrasts his partner's boundaries and authority with his mother's total lack of them. He can sometimes get furious about the difficulties this overly loving mother has saddled him with to date. It is one thing to see what went wrong and why. It is another thing to learn, with great difficulty and often somewhat forcibly, in adulthood what you should have been taught as a child through play and with your mother's milk.

On closer inspection, the father was perhaps the only one who did his 'educational' work correctly. He was often absent owing to his work and did little with his son. In this sense, Chris missed some alliance, camaraderie, and this third party's mediating intervention. On the other hand, he recognises that he also rejected or undermined the father's function himself.

He was helped in this by a mother who was not always loyal to her husband. Perhaps most important for the child's psychological development is not the parent's love for the child but the parents' love for each other. Indulging the child too much seems to form a 'vacancy' within the parental couple with the fatal attraction of a black hole. Willy nilly, the child is sucked into it, with all its consequences for individuation and sexuality.

Chris played *jeux interdits* (forbidden games) with his sister for many years. Many things played a role in these derailments in combination—the mother who offered few boundaries and the father whose authority was challenged. There was a game of attraction and repulsion between brother and sister, a peekaboo of who wields the sceptre/phallus. Outside, the (paternal) law wields the only power. If the law does not work sufficiently, the law of the jungle comes to the fore. The law is, therefore, a friend that protects us from ourselves and others. Otherwise, we are defenceless, at the mercy of the game of will and whim.

In reality, this power element manifested itself in many of Chris's relationships. One moment, he was lord and master. The model for this was a Flamenco dancer he once saw perform in front of a room filled mainly with (fascinated) women. The next moment, he felt himself prey to the omnipotence of his mother/sister, the woman who could castrate him mercilessly.

His sister often called him an idiot or an 'empty head'. He laughed a lot at the joke about men having too little blood volume to simultaneously supply both the erect penis and the brain with sufficient oxygen. Chasing your dick is certainly no fun if it mainly means that the woman (mother) has you by your dick.

Once these themes, object relations, and the corresponding transfers had been sufficiently analysed, Chris steered towards reducing the frequency of his appointments. For several years, he came roughly monthly. From the 'news', he immediately picked out the relevant/the symptomatic. We worked on these loose ends where necessary.

Working through issues is a long process that involves ups and downs and varying degrees of success. The most persistent concerns remained his frustrations at work. He struggled to accept paternal authority and had trouble exercising it. A rebellious child prodigy wanting to play, create, and, in search of phallic affirmation, display his products as showpieces, he felt repeatedly disrespected, short-changed, belittled, and knocked back. He kept striving for a (perfectly succinct) synopsis of his problems. He ended up with these words: 'I am craving admiration, and I am constantly frustrated and irate because of its lack. This makes me a nuisance to myself and others'. We were able to laugh aloud when I complimented him and referred to Freddy Heineken and Sören Kierkegaard, who had 'He Brew' and 'In-Dividu', respectively, on their tombstones. Remember Shakespeare's *brevity is the soul of wit*?

It is sometimes said that Freudian psychoanalysis reduces and that Jungian analysis amplifies. When one has bedroom problems, it is definitely more helpful to relate this to Mum and Dad, but referring to Zeus and Hera can be (more) comforting. Of course, the one option does not exclude the other.

He is trying to 'downsize' now. The sustained effort allows him to find more peace and contentment with his now all-too-real achievements and accomplishments: a solid relationship with all the trimmings, three children, a managerial position as an engineer, and a mansion wholly redesigned and renovated by himself, with a garden at the back that could carry his paper boats out to sea. He seems to have passed the Cape of Good Hope (of castration) and can now better enjoy such 'little' things.

## Simon—Marlboro Man

This smooth, boyish man, in his late 40s, comes for outpatient psychotherapy because of 'some kind of depression'. He consulted his GP for this, who prescribed antidepressants, but to no avail. Spontaneously, he says he has been anxious and nervous since childhood. He was also depressed for the first time over a decade ago. He studied sociology but has always worked in the media.

Simon married Stefanie after a six-year courtship. They stayed together. Although he had recently come out of another relationship and planned to stay single for a while, he has 'stuck' with Stefanie 'from day one'. I am reminded of Victor Hugo's saying: *Qu'est-ce que des amants? Ce sont des nouveau-nés* (What are lovers? They are newborns).

The couple have two little sons. Both have experienced severe health problems. Partly because of this, the couple has grown apart. They have not had any sexual contact 'since forever'. Stefanie finally left him for another partner:

'A real uppercut'. He took care of the children, and, after his wife's affair ended, she returned (at least to take up her parental role) to the marital home. They are not divorced but sleep separately, and each leads their own life: 'The children must not suffer'.

Simon is the younger of two. His parents had children late in life. He describes his father as a very *petit* man who worked as a self-employed shoe-maker. He was said to be anxious, insecure, and well-behaved. Simon speaks somewhat disdainfully of several opportunities his father would not have taken. Simon's mother 'never liked me'. She lived for Simon's older brother. 'I used not to see that. I was used to always coming second.'

He further describes his mother as a rather self-centred and domineering woman. She appears friendly but has a 'difficult character' and is 'on the hysterical side'. She is also said to have exhibitionist tendencies: 'She liked to undress'. A pivotal scene occurs when the mother ostentatiously exposes her breasts in front of the father in the presence of both sons. They embarrassedly giggle away their erotic titillation, but, for Simon, this image is still etched in his memory. He believes it has left him with a weakness for female beauty. 'I am a real boob man.'

Over the years, Simon has accumulated a veritable 'feminatheque' of top-less women and believes he has a voyeuristic tendency from this scene. In his relationships, he does everything to please his partner, sexually and otherwise. 'I am a real show-off.' This excessive 'doing his best' also manifests in other areas of his life and activities.

As a child, he was mischievous and fun-loving. He did not like going to kindergarten. It depended on whether the teacher was 'a dear' or not. 'I needed warmth.' He was always nervous and only found his 'role' in secondary school. He was then in 'a class of jerks'. Simon started smoking and rebelling and adopted the attitude of a 'tough guy'. This image has only begun to crack in recent years. He makes a strong case that quitting smoking did no good. It is as if, by doing so, he has lost something of the 'Marlboro man'.

Simon came to me twice a week for about five years. He installed himself on the sofa swiftly and entirely of his own accord. Free association never seemed to be a problem for him. There was a kind of *'jouissance blabla'*, which he seemed to enjoy. It felt as if he was happy to lay down in my arms/ on the couch to satisfy himself at my breast orally.

It was about his mother for many years. In his account, she appeared as a rather self-centred woman, married, with little conviction, to a not-very-mas-culine figure. She seemed to constantly seek attention from other men (including her sons), towards whom she could often show herself surprisingly lustful. She especially favoured Simon's older brother, and he always felt second-best.

Simon was separation-anxious from childhood, feeling more or less con-stantly 'lost'. His fear of going to school and difficulty standing his ground there (especially in the playground) were never taken up with him or understood by either parent. Things did not improve until he started using an extensive and eloquent vocabulary in adolescence. His verbosity allowed him to 'dick' (out) like the best of them. He also looked to connect with burly fellows and pulled himself up out of an uncertain predicament by clouds of cigarette smoke (the 'heavy kind': Blue Johnson and Green Michel) and with his hair.

He had a whole series of girlfriends and he could wax lyrical about how much he enjoyed tantric sex, where he could keep himself virtually immobile for hours in their moist heat. Nothing could give him greater pleasure than putting a lot of work into and being completely in sync with their waves of orgasm. On closer inspection, he always needed a 'buddy' with whom he could feel wordlessly connected.

There were often two women involved simultaneously: one with whom he had an official relationship, who could offer him security and stability, and one with whom he could be more of an adventurous rake and bad boy. From his adolescent years, he was never once *without* a woman. Although he did well everywhere in terms of his professional life and made it quite far, his career seemed to be the least of his worries.

Instead, Simon was a *soldier of love*. In his analysis, he often returned to a line from a Joe Cocker song: 'You don't know what love is; I will show you what love is'. Whether as a partner, a friend, or a father, he was a paragon of empathy, attunement, emotional care, and other caring. Anger at what he had missed in terms of maternal love was then (besides identification with the other-equal) a significant driving force for making love a verb.

During his analysis, he managed to end a fake status and then divorce his wife for real anyway. He had realised, 'I have a mother who is not a mother and a wife who is not a wife'. Why remain stuck in a structurally unsatisfactory situation?

There was a significant shift in his sexual experience. He became more interested in buttocks and vaginas, went through a period of brothel visits, which revolved more around his desires, and experimented with cybersex. In this way, he explored and discovered more of his sexuality and abandoned a very idealising attitude towards the opposite sex.

He made a bold career move, leaving the security of steady work and embarking on a new phase in his professional life by moving into the health-care sector.

The grand finale of his therapy was an intense infatuation with a much younger co-worker who was initially very seductive towards him. Blind to the fact that they were over a generation apart in age, they plunged into romantic engagements and initiatives. It felt like 'first love' (again).

*It takes two to tango.* Careful analysis revealed that there seemed to be an unconscious 'match' at play between the two. At first, they seemed to be the answer to each other's needs. Only when the girl suddenly, unexpectedly, but mostly coldly, began to reject him could Simon dwell on the depth of these feelings. An old wound of unrequited first love for his mother opened, and extensive mourning could be done for the loss of this first love object.

Initially with some inhibition, Simon eventually started work as a therapist. He seemed fearful that I would blow back or criticise him for this. He started treating the psychotherapy session more as a supervision opportunity. As soon as he realised this, he decided to quit and start further training.

## Frederik—How Strong Is the Lone Cyclist

This 30-something came to consult following the death of his former psychiatrist. Some five years earlier, he had consulted this colleague, and the latter had promptly, after barely one consultation, prescribed dexamphetamine sulphate for his 'ADD'. Frederik called this rather abrupt, 'because we never spoke effectively'.

He has found his general condition deteriorating in recent years. He feels emotionally flattened. 'I never experience bursts of happiness.' He feels 'always on' and says he has no deep sleep. 'I am never delighted.' He talks at once about his personality. 'I can't talk, bottle up, avoid; everything is processed internally. Quiet people have a loud mind!'

He has two bachelor's degrees, works in the computer industry, and has lived with Sylvia, a slightly younger teacher, for three years. Fortunately, she is very extraverted, as he calls himself demure. 'We fit together perfectly.'

'My parents are still(!) together.' He describes them as 'sweet but emotionally absent'; there is little depth. He describes his mother as very caring. She can show feelings but not talk about them. There is an immediate story about the father. He lost his mother when he was barely six. He is not very communicative and had to go to work very young. He describes his father as old-fashioned and insecure. To Frederik's mind, his father never stood by him. He was relaxed at home until he heard his father's motorbike announcing his return from work in the evening. From then on, it was like, 'Pay attention!' and 'Forward, march!' Frederik often retreated to his room and sat behind a screen playing games. His father complained about this, a concealed polarisation ensued, and they became increasingly distant and hostile. Two younger brothers were 'allowed anything by father' and could do nothing wrong in his eyes. He has little connection with them. 'It was kind of every man for himself.'

At first, Frederik describes himself as a 'very normal child'—playing sports, having friends. However, he often felt he did not belong from secondary school onwards. There was a lot of insecurity. 'I missed a sounding board.' He threw himself into cycling, where he trained hard (but alone). In groups, he had to adapt to the pace of others. Then, he preferred to train alone: he raced against the clock, going 'to extremes. It was a real outlet'. When he started competing, his relationship with his father came under even more pressure. In his father's eyes, it was an expensive hobby, and he thought

Frederik should rather be working. When he started winning races, his father gave no reaction. Frederik's mother came to support him. 'She was my rock.'

From the first session, some verses from a song by the Dutch singer-songwriter Boudewijn de Groot came to mind: 'How strong is the lonely cyclist/ who bent over his handlebars against the wind/forces his way through'. According to Wilfred Bion, such incursions can result from unconscious communication within the analytical pair and require (in his terms) an 'act of faith' (in the unconscious) to produce them in due course. Frederik could immediately relate to this, and, thus, the tone of our collaboration was set.

From the start, Frederik showed himself to be reflective and motivated in the weekly psychotherapy. He diligently (figuratively) 'jotted down' insights in advance and, in the following session, he immediately picked up the thread to explore it further. I concur with Jacques Lacan, who refers to an analysand with a 't' (*analysant*) because of this (ideally) active attitude.

Initially, however, Frederik thought he was born with a form of autism spectrum disorder and was constitutionally condemned to a socially restricted life. Much has already been written about autistic disorders by psychoanalysts, but a whole range of psychopathology is situated under this banner. Thanks to evolving knowledge on the subject, late diagnoses of autism spectrum disorder are being made more and more often nowadays. It is, then, regarded mainly as a neurocognitive developmental disorder, causing a patient's 'computer' to work atypically. It is a harsh but invisible (as well as fearfully/frenetically hidden by the patient and often misunderstood for both reasons) condition that the patient suffers 24/7. It can lead to burnout-like exhaustion symptoms and can even end in suicidality and euthanasia requests. What does—from the margin—the bell of a Gaussian curve look like? Isn't it a barely surveyable mountain of 'normality', which you look up to as a statistical deviant because of its impracticability?

However, it soon emerged that, initially, he was a calm little boy who managed to make many friends in kindergarten, for example, and win many a girl's heart. As an aside, kindergarten may safely be called a scene of passion, for it is often forgotten (or repressed) by those involved and those around them how much amorous and hostile tempers can flare at that stage of life!

He realised how significantly his father impacted his emotional and social development. Unlike with his mother and wife, he clashed with his father's Gestalt: a malevolent rather than benevolent outside world. Meanwhile, he gradually became entrenched in his (upstairs) room and only got 'outside' via computers/gaming and sports. Various metaphors passed in review. These included the 'bunker' he had built in response to numerous unexpected blasts from his father and an armour of numbness and indifference he had donned from childhood. Both hindered his ability to establish a deeper emotional connection with others. He had thrived with regard to intellectual and sporting achievements, but much less on a social and relational level. It gradually became clear that Sylvia had taken over the torch from his mother, but she offered much more 'nourishment' emotionally/communicatively. After all, the mother could gasp and snap when he wanted to say things she would rather not hear. Frederik had a great appetite, both with his partner and with me.

Fortunately, not all psychotherapy is complex and prolonged labour. With Frederik, there was soon some pleasure and enjoyment. The many details and anecdotes that further substantiated the described pattern came up in weekly torrents, and, in his actual life, too, his communicative potential broadened with equal pace, and he sporadically even managed to emerge as an esteemed, because humorous, entertainer—at least according to Sylvia.

A straightforward psychoanalytic therapist does not let himself be 'caught' by this striking prima facie progression. He is, as it were, on high alert for signs of a negative (rather than idealising) father transference. Sooner or later, he is bound to fall short, empathically or otherwise. This offers both 'parties' the opportunity to experience in vivo how Frederik emotionally and (inter) actively deals with such frustrations so that his profoundly ingrained problem with his father becomes a living reality within psychotherapy and can also be worked on, with varying degrees of success.

### Renée—Victim of Too Much Success

This teacher, in her mid-30s, was referred for more thorough psychotherapy after initial admission to a PWGH service. She has led a hectic life for many years and never questioned it. After all, nothing bothered her, and she was unaware that anything was wrong. After the birth of her fourth child, however, she had suffered some hyperventilation and 'balance disorders'. She had been physically investigated several times, but nothing was found. A few months before, her husband suffered a brain haemorrhage for which urgent surgery was required. For quite some time, he still showed severe residual neurological symptoms. Initial confusion about delirious phenomena gave way to a frontal syndrome characterised by disinhibition, loss of decorum, and character change. 'He was not my husband anymore. Our relationship became almost unliveable.'

For quite a while, Renée remained extremely active: she kept working full-time, looked after the children, including managing their various leisure activities, and went back and forth to the hospital several times a day. On the other hand, internally, she felt more and more anxiety and insecurity. Meanwhile, according to Renée, her husband is 95 per cent his old self again. He is still a bit more short-tempered than before but is working hard again. When he fell a few weeks earlier and suffered some superficial head injuries, she panicked a lot and feared another catastrophe. She is now suffering the reaction to the difficult period. There are nightmares and flashbacks. She sleeps a lot and, despite this, she has a tremendous and persistent fatigue that contrasts sharply with her customary vigour and work ethic. She is not the same person anymore and now realises she has burnt the candle at both ends for far too long. 'I went way over a limit without realising it.'

Renée is the third of five children. Her father has a corporate managerial position, which means he is away a lot and often abroad for somewhat more extended periods. At home, he is sweet, warm, and involved. He read bedtime stories and played board games with the children. According to Renée, her mother is a lovely, concerned mother who was always available: 'A real mum'. She did homework together with the children, and they baked pancakes together.

Renée was always a very easy-going and carefree child. She loved going to school and was always top of her class. She had many friends, learned to play several instruments at music school, was in the youth movement, and went horse riding. In her adolescence, she hardly rebelled. After failing to finish university, she studied to be a teacher. She is used to being a sunshine girl who can handle all difficulties effortlessly and with a smile. Now, in recent months, she has been bumping up against limitations she cannot cope with and almost does not recognise herself. 'I feel so weak!'

Renée was in inpatient psychotherapy with us for just under a year. Since then, she has been going to weekly outpatient meetings with a psychologist-psychotherapist and comes to me monthly for psychiatric and process counselling. She has scrutinised her life history from top to bottom and bottom to top and can now come to only one conclusion: 'I can't deal with the fact that there are things I can't deal with'.

Renée experienced a very happy, loving, and carefree childhood and youth. She was liked and accepted by everyone and always received high praise everywhere. In a way, she became a victim of her success. She cannot stand failure and cannot stand losing. She was always a winner who could do magic. She was often told: 'How you manage all that!' The fact that things do not keep going effortlessly and/or brilliantly is a harsh reality that she was unprepared for.

Renée works part-time, looking after her four children just fine and holding her own alongside a husband who sometimes plays with the children but has otherwise wholly given up on his role as father. He is regularly angry, and she has to take extra care of the children. She fruitlessly seeks recognition for her weakness and fatigue, which she feels no one listens to. With these hidden problems, she feels stubbornly left out in the cold. 'That I have to go to therapists for that!'

## Jane—the Possibility of an Island

Jane is a 30-something single woman who was referred after several admissions (including to psychiatric hospitals) following yet another suicide attempt and because of lingering and severe depressive symptoms. She is the fourth in a family of five children. Several family members were hospitalised and/or otherwise treated for depression.

Her mother is described as a chronically depressed woman. She is dead to touch, can enjoy little or nothing, and is very frugal and prudish. She has always leaned heavily on Jane emotionally, so Jane had to be sturdy, gutsy, and sensible from childhood. Her father is described as a sexist 'womaniser' who allegedly cheated on her mother on several occasions. Even in old age, he still repeatedly expresses his sexual needs. 'Hopefully, the home help doesn't have too many curves. Otherwise, he won't be able to keep his hands off.' Father was also hardly involved in parenting but did make all kinds of sexual innuendos in her adolescence and interfered in an overly sexualising way with her however 'innocent' puppy-love. Furthermore, he is hot-tempered, authoritarian, and domineering in his actions, and she experiences his emotional understanding as being very limited, if not non-existent. As far as she was concerned, the parents had a loveless relationship. 'I never saw any sign of warmth between them.'

Jane has minimal social contact. During a volatile relationship, she deliberately pushed for pregnancy and she cares for her only daughter as a single parent. For fear of burdening her daughter emotionally, she did have the courage to allow her to attend boarding school, improving their relationship quality at weekends and in the holidays.

Jane must constantly keep herself straight and upright by doing arithmetic related to all sorts of things. Thus, she tries to 'watch her step' and hold on to the branches of trees, so to speak, to avoid sinking into an inner abyss. There is also great rational control, holding off all feelings. This is then 'compensated' by a very active dream life. She can often remember her dreams very well and gradually developed the ability to analyse them and extract meaningful content from them.

Jane has now been in psychotherapy for more than a decade. She went through two episodes of inpatient psychotherapy that lasted about a year each time. She was then balancing on the brink of suicide. Much care was needed to ensure her survival, and, at times, even support of her vital functions (as in physical medicine) was required to continue the psychotherapy operation. Since then, she has attended face-to-face psychotherapy with a psychoanalyst twice a week and comes to me monthly for psychiatric and psychoanalytic process counselling.

Jane works part-time as a child carer and eagerly participates in what goes on between mothers and their newborns. She sometimes identifies more with one side of a couple than the other. She missed a lot with her mother and was inversely parented by her. Her mother, then, has something of the dead mother that Andre Green, for instance, talks about. She was, as it were, a black sun, emitting neither light nor warmth and instead sucking in all energy like a black hole.

By now, there have been innumerable dreams in which Jane has to clean up other people's 'shit'. She often comes across dirty or otherwise unusable toilets so that there is nowhere she can be at 'ease' and 'do her business'. Instead of solid ground underfoot, she feels she is above an abyss or on a hole's only half-closed 'lid'. Thus, she regularly finds herself in 'free-fall'—the unthinkable fear or nameless horror of Donald Winnicott or Wilfred Bion, respectively. Like Baron Von Munchhausen, she tries pulling herself out of the quagmire by her hair. She often uses addition, counting rhymes, or simply counts elapsing seconds.

Such obsessional thoughts offer her a footing, but, unlike the transitional ones, they are not living or animated but dead or autistic objects to which she clings without being able to open up more symbolic horizons of meaning or significance. She misses the sun and warmth and seeks out various southern islands every holiday break to recharge her batteries.

For many years, Jane has had a boyfriend who turns out to be a kind of father figure to her daughter but with whom she remains emotionally and sexually hungry. He is a conservative man who is very rational and—to a sexist extent—installs himself in the traditional division of roles, evoking reminiscences of her father. The maternal environment of the therapeutic relationships that nurtured her inner life was particularly beneficial for Jane.

Classical dream analysis played a massive role in interpretive work. Several dreams would come up each session, and she became adept at deciphering their hidden messages. For all these years, she took a maintenance dose of antidepressants, but her case may still mainly concern a primary or anaclitic depression related to an (emotionally) absent mother. These depressive feelings can be chemically mitigated, but they have the right to exist and should be acknowledged, recognised, and understood as such. Psychotherapy can be seen as a protracted process of working through steady and reliable therapeutic encounters from which a more true and vibrant self can grow.

## Britt—a Good Connection

This 30-something working in the care sector was referred after she had already experienced six admissions in seven years because of what she says is 'psychosis and depression'. The first time, she experienced 'postpartum psychosis' after the birth of her first child. On closer inspection, this state was mainly characterised by massive and catastrophic anxieties, as she feared going mad and losing her mind. A confused twilight state and disorders of consciousness and impending disintegration were in the zenith. There was excessive religious preoccupation, and Britt felt surrounded by the spectres of deceased people acting as 'guardian angels'.

Since then, she has experienced a similar condition several times, each time requiring hospitalisation. However, this troubled state clears once she is placed in a caring environment. There are psychiatric antecedents for depression in several family members on her mother's side. Habitually, she describes herself as very fragile. However, she manages to hide this behind a hefty and gritty façade.

Britt is the middle of three children. Her parents divorced when she was seven years old. Mother is an administrative clerk. She experienced 'moments of warmth' with her, but, because of severe alcohol addiction, material, educational, and affective neglect was the norm. Britt then had to look after her mother instead of vice versa. She felt 'damaged' by her mother.

Father also has an alcohol problem, but 'I can count on him'. She has a much better relationship with him. Between the ages of 10 and 16, an incestuous relationship developed with her older brother. 'I sought closeness and affection from him', but this degenerated into the sexual. 'However, I enjoyed his love, attention and gentleness.' She lacks this dimension in her relationship with her husband, whom she has known since the age of 16. On the other hand, she struggles with sexual contact. She is afraid of men. She also fears that her children would be victims of abuse.

She had an inpatient psychotherapy admission of several months. Here, a different and better foundation was laid for what has now been several years of continuous outpatient psychotherapy. Still, many hardly realise the disastrous impact of alcoholic parents on child development. There is a beautiful and enlightening website, Adult Children of Alcoholics, where expected consequences are clearly described. A mixture of parentification and varying degrees of neglect inevitably accompany it. There are acute conflicts between anger and anxiety, and feelings of loyalty complicate separation–individuation. There is an unnerving cycle of hope (in abstinence) and disillusionment (in relapse), which creates a permanent stress factor and source of insecurity. Attachment problems are pervasive and go hand in hand with impaired or immature mentalising abilities.

Apart from a possible constitutional vulnerability, Britt is a textbook example of this. She was taking a low dose of an atypical antipsychotic continuously. Occasionally, this had to be increased for a few days to avoid an impending crisis and/or admission. She feels understood and supported by her psychotherapist and makes more or less use of her psychotherapist as a kind of developmental object according to her evolving needs.

Integration of split-off (abandonment) anger reduces the disruptive effect that such 'unbound' aggression exerts on her psyche. In this context, she often talks about implosion as opposed to explosion. The various themes and aspects that play a role in her psychopathology come up alternately: abandonment and neglect; fear and insecurity; anger and anxiety; the father who was too absent because he never actually interfered; becoming entangled in an incestuous relationship with her brother, which has to be understood mainly as two children in distress clinging to each other.

She transitioned from working in the care sector to education during her therapy. Her marriage, which began as a care-based father–child relationship, evolved into a partner relationship on an equal footing in which the sexual also had more of a role. It cannot be ruled out that she will keep the therapeutic relationship open for quite some time. She comes much more infrequently, and often it suffices for her to notice that I am online with her in an attuned way and that, in other words, we manage to maintain a 'good connection'.

## Carmen—the Asylum Seeker

This young adult woman requested admission herself after being discharged against advice following a conflict in another psychiatric hospital. She had been in treatment there for five years, with ups and downs. Since her first suicide attempt at 18, she had been hospitalised almost constantly in various (including university) psychiatric settings.

Carmen is the younger of two. Her father is a civil servant. He was almost always drunk, strict, and demanding towards Carmen. She received little or no support or validation from him. Under the influence of alcohol, he was also sometimes somewhat sexually transgressive. The mother is a blue-collar worker and is described as psychologically unstable. Carmen had to care for her mother and only received 'false love' from her. If there were problems, Carmen had to call the police or the doctor herself. 'If we were sick, we were punished and had to stay in our room.'

Carmen often hoped that her sister and she would be taken away and that her parents would divorce. They were not allowed to talk about anything. She communicated with her sister through notes they exchanged at the table. The atmosphere at home was unsafe and unfriendly. There was neither warmth nor affection. She sat in her room a lot, curled up in a ball under the blankets. On top of that, she retreated into a fantasy world with imaginary boyfriends a lot.

She was a very anxious child, and psychological help was suggested by the school medical service, which her parents refused. Between the ages of 6 and 12, she (like her older sister) was sexually abused by an uncle on her mother's side who took them up to the attic and silenced them with death threats. It only stopped when Carmen started menstruating. She also developed severe anorexia around that period. 'I didn't want to become a woman.' She also began exhibiting self-harming behaviour.

In her adolescence, she had a partner with a severe drug addiction who molested her. She was also briefly married to an abusive partner. She left both of them by going to a refuge. She had several short relationships 'to avoid being alone'. When they wanted to 'move on', she dropped out. On admission, she is in a relationship with a man who was also a victim of sexual abuse and is in psychiatric treatment. He is gentle, respectful, and understanding. With him, she finds some security for the first time.

Psychotherapy, unfortunately, is not always a success story. There is, classically, the possibility of an adverse therapeutic reaction. For example, the patient may be unconsciously intent on flooring the therapist. They then choose to let illness 'triumph' over health. Often, this is framed within a narcissistic issue to belittle or degrade the therapist. Being alpha and omega oneself leaves little room for the therapist to play a significant role. This can be called a death drive or primitive envy/aversion in which the good breast is destroyed not because it does not provide but—on the contrary—because it does provide vital nourishment. The patient cannot stomach the fact that the (source of) goodness is external, much less that they would depend on it. They would prefer to drop dead than to recognise their own needy or distressed state.

On the one hand, Carmen was cooperative throughout her treatment. She tried to tell her story, making constructive use of expressive therapy and using collages around various themes to outsmart resistance, as it were, and involuntarily bring the patient to 'deep' feelings or sensitivities. Of course, this presupposes a sufficiently active therapist who 'translates' signifiers in the context of the life history and what takes place (metaphorically and counter-transferentially) within the therapeutic encounter.

On the other hand, Carmen's early-childhood/'oral' needs were such that she insisted on intensive and exclusive care, even in the context of very persistent acting-out behaviour, time and again. With each new patient that joined, sibling rivalry immediately arose, and relapse was challenging to discuss and correct. With Carmen, the main obstacle to therapeutic progress was regression. Period.

A safety net is not a hammock, and a couch is not for sleeping on. Within any psychoanalytic treatment, regression is necessary to reach the point of fixation and act on it 'in vivo' and not 'in vitro'. Regression is at the service of the ego and the service of therapy. It provides a lived insight within the therapeutic relationship that distinguishes itself from mere cognitive/rational insight or theory.

All attempts at progression and resocialisation failed. Carmen did not seem to want to grow and become independent. The hospital, with its holding and facilitating (maternal) environment, was a place for her not to grow up but to stay small, fill her bottomless 'hole', and shelter from an outside world full of sexual and other dangers and predators.

Despite sustained attunement to these understandable fears and feelings, and although this was worked on interpretively ad nauseam, any attempt to let go and become more independent led to escalating acting-out behaviour and 'suicidality'. Several auto-intoxications then landed her in an emergency department. Afterwards, it was almost back to square one each time.

As there was no breakthrough, Carmen was referred to another psychiatric hospital with more social-psychiatric assets/pseudopods than ours: a location on the outskirts of a city centre, a day clinic, assisted living on campus, and psychiatric care at home. She has also been in treatment there for many years.

I learned from a close colleague that she successively went through the various departments with optimal treatment durations of 3 months, 12 months, and 36 months, respectively. There, the same pattern has emerged. The patient brightens up as long as the end is not in sight. She dresses up, goes shopping, and steps out into the world at weekends.

After several attempts at assisted living failed, and in the face of imminent discharge from the hospital, she attempted suicide again while in lodgings with relatives in another region. From the local general hospital, she was referred to a psychiatric hospital there. It is one of those psychiatric dinosaurs that, until decades ago, still acted as an asylum. What has happened to the days when many patients could, and were allowed to, stay there, sometimes for the rest of their life?

## Brigitte—from Persecution Fears to Underdogs

This 30-something woman was referred for inpatient psychotherapy because of depressive symptoms that emerged some two years earlier. The trigger was several miscarriages and an ectopic pregnancy after she had already undergone several in vitro fertilisation treatments. In reality, she had greatly longed for a cosy family with several children. In addition, her husband's own business went bankrupt, and she says she took all this very much to heart.

Brigitte is the youngest of three children. She says that her parents are rather strict. The father is said to be on the aggressive side and is regularly violent. She is afraid of him. The mother is initially sketched as a sweet, helpful woman. Brigitte is married and has two children, both of whom are said to be hyperactive. She worked in the care sector until the birth of her children. She is said to have been a sociable, cheerful, and vibrant child. There were tensions around her choice of study, though, with Brigitte wanting to be a hairdresser but not being allowed by her parents.

Based on these initial anamnestic data and her history from the introductory interview, one might deduce that an admission of, say, three months should more than suffice to allow Brigitte to recover her equilibrium, lay the foundations for a further therapeutic relationship, and start outpatient psychotherapy in which underlying feelings and sensitivities can be worked on.

On closer inspection, however, the initial data were highly misleading. They described only the surface of a false self. It soon became apparent that Brigitte was 'terrified' of her parents. Her mother lacked empathy and could instead rage at her in an ugly and reproachful manner. She demanded that she stop her treatment as soon as possible and keep silent about the past. Only after many years of therapy was she able to admit that she had also been a victim of sexual abuse by her father. Brigitte's father also opposed the treatment and, despite his daughter's age, still regularly hit her if she disobeyed him or dared to speak out.

From childhood, Brigitte was very scared. She anxiously tried to comply with what her parents expected of her. She had been sexually abused for years by her maternal grandfather as well as, sporadically, by her brother and a family friend. The latter had lured her to the garden house. He threatened murder and manslaughter if she spoke and, when she tried to flee, he chased her, brandishing garden tools. 'He wanted to bash my head in.'

She constantly felt abandoned and abused as a child. Even in her marriage, she was often alone with all her worries, given her husband's busy self-employment. In the first months of her clinical psychotherapy treatment, her husband left her for another woman.

While she had enjoyed several years of a reasonably happy family, she now had to turn back to her parents for help. Materially and logistically (household and financial support, childcare), they were accommodating. Still, on the other hand, they eagerly used this renewed dependence to control her movements: they confiscated her bank card, she was no longer allowed to drive her car, and they were constantly making things difficult in connection with the hospital's curfew. We often had to keep her in because of life-threatening crises, and this was thwarted or sabotaged by the parents, who saw nothing positive in our approach and accused us of only being greedy for money.

Brigitte struggled with severe feelings of abandonment, rage, and depression. She injured herself so persistently that, for months, she ended up in emergency rooms several times a week to have her injuries stitched up. Meanwhile, she was also haunted day and night by post-traumatic re-experiences, which often drove her to suicide attempts and the emergency room.

It took a lot of work to get her to the point where she no longer allowed herself to be annihilated by everyone but dared to show her teeth and bite when necessary. Step by step, she managed to regain lost ground: she found a place to live, was able to get behind the wheel of her car, and went into day treatment. After treatments that included four years of ups and downs and episodes of full and day hospitalisation, she has now been on an outpatient basis for about three years.

Both sons have since come to live with her. She volunteers several times a week. In one of her posts, she was exploited for a time as a free maid-of-all-work by a single career woman and mother of three. With the necessary fear of retaliation and bleeding heart for the children, who she felt were affectionately wronged, she escaped from the clutches of this mother superior.

She sees a very supportive and caring female GP weekly and comes for monthly psychiatric consultations. It remains a struggle to keep her head above water, but, within the therapeutic space, there is safety and enjoyment to which undertones, witticisms, and the occasional hearty laugh testify.

## William—Clint Eastwood's Son

After a childhood from which a lot of rebellion and behavioural problems, in particular, have been retained, William developed a history of years of lingering polytoxicomania (heroin, cocaine, cannabis, and amphetamines) and alcohol abuse for which there had already been multiple admissions to psychiatric hospitals and drug-free therapeutic communities. He was referred from one of the latter for inpatient psychotherapy. It is felt that 'underlying problems' need to be worked on. He is, at that point, weaned and 'clean'.

William immediately talks about his father, who died by suicide. He describes his father as a demanding, authoritarian, sometimes violent man. He represented a *boys don't cry*-like macho culture. 'If you are in pain or grief, you should chop wood in the garden.' With some admiration and sympathy, on the other hand, he calls his father a Flemish Clint Eastwood. William was still in his classroom when his father became the school head-master. 'There was nowhere for me to escape him then!'

William is the middle of three sons. The eldest brother is said to have been 'broken' by his father, and the youngest is gay. According to William, the mother is a caring woman who would always have lived to serve his father and produces a lot of 'blabla'. It is not the only derogatory expression about women we hear in the course of our conversations. Around the age of 13, William experienced a traumatising training weekend during which he was locked up and sexually abused by a sports teacher. It was a man with whom he had got on well until then and with whom he had felt safe and supported. This left him with a great distrust of, and hostility towards, those in authority: 'In the end, they are all fat bastards'.

William has been feeling—excessively since then—very afraid of bonding, of being known, of being dependent, and of being vulnerable. He is terrified of closeness, friendship, and love. 'It all brings nothing but misery.' If some-one gets too close, he freaks out. He alienates them and soon gets a dirty feeling 'that I can only get rid of with all kinds of drugs'. There has been a massive flight into substance abuse from puberty onwards. It frames him in a negativist/oppositional attitude towards society but mainly aims to flatten all brain functions and completely clear his head. Indeed, as is so often the case with trauma patients, William suffers from failing repression or, as he says, not being able to forget.

William was only in clinical psychotherapy for about three months, which felt extremely long because, from the start, he wanted to be discharged, against advice. 'It's like a prison here.' He had a cool, roguish attitude in the group, constantly mocking and making snide comments about the therapists' pomposity there. In individual contacts, too, he was initially very giggly at every attempt at psychotherapeutic rapprochement. Whenever he went out, he returned drunk. He then refused to stay in the room, although this is one of the ward rules for such problem behaviour. However, he felt too confined and needed to be able to 'break out'. 'I can't help it!'

A sufficient portion of humour and playfulness was needed to thaw him a little in the contact. Through a comment here and there, he then opened up for a while. This was mostly about his father's harsh attitude and how he had missed 'empathy and affection' from his father. The (in this case, sexual) pre-dator invariably chooses a 'weak' victim, and William felt very embarrassed that he had allowed himself to be 'done' like this. He was furious with himself for having 'let himself be done like a sissy'. However, what had occurred on the weekend in question was only expressed in veiled terms.

By applying for jobs while admitted and having been able to sell himself well for a great job, he was discharged far too early as far as we were con-cerned. The main result of his admission was that he could establish the foundations of a trusting relationship. It ensured that he came to me (albeit irregularly) for about five years. He worked continuously in well-paid technical positions, being 'on the road' a lot and predominantly 'his own boss'.

A methadone dependency had installed itself, though, which was maintained by a slightly older female addiction specialist. He has been in a steady, cohabiting relationship with her for several years, which he calls emotionally satisfying. She is said to be very loving and understanding, and this is despite brief moments of relapse into heroin use. They are accompanied by outbursts of sexual aversion towards his partner as well as sexual acting-out in which he says he behaves like an 'arsehole' towards the stranger girls he manages to snare with his unapproachable *cool*.

Tears sometimes come into his eyes when he confesses such states to me. 'It is as if a monster takes over inside me.' He feels the link with what he went through with the perpetrator, but how this works still eludes him. After he let slip in an unguarded moment how meaningful our conversations were to him, he hasn't reappeared. 'For each man kills the thing he loves' is a quote by the famous Irish writer and homosexual Oscar Wilde that once featured on one of his T-shirts. I thought it was a remarkable reference for a son of Dirty Harry. Hopefully, sooner or later, we will find out how meaningful the quote is for his psychodynamics.

## Magda—the Storming of the Balcony

This office worker in her mid-40s was referred after several admissions to a PWGH service but also to other psychiatric hospitals because of lingering depressive symptoms. There, to a greater or lesser extent, she became entangled in idealising infatuation and dependency towards female therapists whom she even started stalking over time. During her last admission, she got to know a much older fellow patient for whom she left her husband.

Magda complains of highly fluctuating moods in which she sometimes throws herself enthusiastically and over-actively into a new venture and then falls, 'down and empty', into a hole. After several failed relationships, she married, without much conviction, a man who fully lived up to the norm (of her parents). They have four children. Her husband built a successful career but was very rational and emotionally unavailable. They lived under the same roof, but each led their own life.

She is the youngest of three children and the only daughter. Her father died during Magda's first psychiatric admission. He had a managerial position and was absent, quiet, and closed-minded. She looked up to him because of his intellect and had 'more connection' with him than with her mother. She also calls him 'very loyal': he would never have cheated on her mother. Her mother was a housewife and rather dominant. She saw everything in black and white, was emotionally unavailable, and, according to Magda, had 'no feeling'.

At first, Magda is said to have been a cheerful and upbeat child. However, by her admission, she found it difficult to be happy and had difficulty being alone. During her adolescence, there were many conflicts with her mother, who constantly interfered in everything and viewed everything negatively. She always felt very independent and had very variable—because superficial—contacts. 'I was detached. It was as if I felt nothing.'

In both kindergarten and primary school, there had been teachers to whom Magda became overly attached and for whom she tried to hold a special place. Even when she had her children, she was very attached to her gynaecologist because he was caring and understanding.

She was hospitalised in our clinical psychotherapeutic milieu. She followed several years of full admission, day therapy, outpatient therapy, and repeated re-admission because of depressive relapses and suicidality. More than once, we discussed all this as an almost addictive dependency. In psychiatry, she seemed to have tasted a forbidden fruit whose taste never seemed to leave her. Paraphrasing Shakespeare, *she had eaten from the root that takes the reason prisoner.*

As expected, she developed a fusional and consuming (transference) love for her psychotherapist. She did not want to be one of many patients in line for her but to hold a special place, even in her heart. She clashed and interfered with professional boundaries and challenged the laws and rules I imposed on her as departmental psychiatrist/authority.

Besides ups and downs, framed in a 'mood disorder' (lithium certainly had a stabilising effect in this respect), there was in her a struggle between the rational and the emotional, the progressive and the regressive, the adult and the baby part. On the one hand, she emerged as a co-therapist and spoke out in ward meetings, challenging all kinds of policies. On the other hand, she became, each time, trapped in and overwhelmed by a nostalgic yearning for our ward/environmental mother, embodied mainly by her busty psychologist.

When it was pointed out to her again and again that this scenario repeated itself throughout her life with ever-changing actors and actresses, she gradually got to grips with the deeply oral, early-childhood root of this symptom. It was harrowing, but she got in touch with a kind of vampire inside her, which, with a mixture of love and hate, wanted to sink its teeth into the white and virginal neck/bosom of the psychotherapist, as it were.

Then things slipped into dream material where she penetrated the bedroom and the intimacy of the parental couple. During the day, too, she gradually saw more flashes of, for her, very embarrassing images in which she saw all kinds of people (including her therapists) naked and imagined how they 'did it'. She experienced these as sexual compulsions that contrasted sharply with her virtually non-existent libido.

She attributed the latter to the fact that sexuality seemed taboo in her parental home. It was also related to the fact that she was involved in playing doctor by her older brother as well as to a first negative sexual experience after which she had felt brutalised by the male sex. Recently, her fascination with the female sex, in particular, has been confusing her more and more. 'Could I be attracted to women after all?'

She has now celebrated her tenth year 'outside psychiatry'. On a few occasions, she needed some breakdown assistance for several weeks in a PWGH service. Apart from that, she attends weekly outpatient psychotherapy. Despite this low frequency, deep oral fantasies and anxieties can be discussed in almost Kleinian terms, thanks in part to a lot of dream material. Not only the emotional inaccessibility of her mother but also sibling rivalry and penis envy concerning her older brother are discussed at length. Despite his drinking and failed career, he remains his mother's favourite.

Only at this later stage (and then only in talking) does her sexual life come up in more detail. Besides a critical oral component, a negative Oedipal constellation and an actively conquering/phallic disposition also play an essential role. While she continued to 'stalk' our psychiatric hospital/mother institute and her psychologist for years, this has completely calmed down. After the transference was shifted to me, we could analyse her idealising transference in more detail. A series of unattainable figures had passed through her life, about whom she could dream and fantasise as if they embodied the (promised) land of milk and honey—the ultimate hallucination.

We talked at length about the connection between mourning complicated by love and hate for the primary all-good object and her cyclothymic mood disorder. Moments of emptiness and fulfilment alternated here. Sometimes, there were persecutive fears (a breast that would avenge itself on her) and then depressive anxieties (I bit/destroyed the breast once and for all).

A calm has set in for a year now. She marvels at how long things could have been so turbulent. In retrospect, what was almost a storm in a teacup has quieted. 'What have I been doing all this time!' Only now does she realise how much she has failed as a mother as a result of countless long-term hospitalisations. Like a penitent, she slaves away for her children to make up for the harm done. For their part, they do not cease to present her with the bill repeatedly: a tragic situation in which there are only losers, and not everyone has been made equally wiser.

## Bea—not Genes but Allergens

This 30-something woman comes for outpatient psychotherapy consultations of her own accord.

> Every three weeks, I change for no apparent reason. That screws up a lot. I have trouble letting go. I am a real control freak. This was also a big problem in previous relationships. My husband doesn't like that. I don't take any initiative. I get the same comments from all my partners. However, I grew up in a normal family. Father was a dominant figure. He was a manager and is now in his seventies. Mother was not allowed anything from him. It was later revealed that he had a mistress from when I was three. My parents divorced when I was twenty. I was angry. Why now?

Bea is the youngest of three. In her own words, she had 'an okay childhood'. She had plenty of girlfriends and was always among the 'cool ones' in the class. She had many concentration problems during secondary school, and her grades went downhill. 'I was internally absent.' She was, however, very sporty. Physical exercise calmed her down. 'I have such a bad basic feeling.' She has always liked being alone and travelling worldwide, in adolescence and adulthood. She never had a good relationship with her father. 'Actually, no bond.' She does not feel good with him. She feels anger that is hard to bring home. 'I avoid him. I put up my spines. I set myself up negatively. I wasn't sexually abused, after all!' Spontaneously, Bea explains that her father had a bad childhood. That his parents abused him. The grandmother on her father's side appears coercive and possessive. 'We all have something of our father in us.' He cannot tolerate anything and is very irritable at the slightest thing. Her mother used to be a very social woman and is from a large peasant family. Her marriage changed her greatly. She was often broken down by Bea's father and gradually lost her self-confidence. The father scolded her and made hurtful remarks. He even wanted his spouse to be declared crazy after the divorce. However, he could be very weird himself and was, at times, even physically threatening.

Bea did higher studies and worked for the government. Her current partner has been her best friend for many years, and they have been in a living-apart-together relationship for a year. Now that she is pregnant, they will move in together, but she fears feeling trapped or imprisoned. Her past relationships never lasted longer than this one. She was never enthusiastic and constantly felt like 'leave me alone'. She cannot express herself or let herself go. She always feels more like a spectator than a participant. 'I observe everything.' She struggles with the fact that her husband smokes and drinks. With some embarrassment, she says she prefers fresh, sporty people; her thinking is very black and white here.

One kitten or puppy is not like another. The little animals can be calm or anxious, close or distant, depending on the litter they come from. They cannot tell, of course, but what they have experienced in their earliest development sets the tone for how they stand in the world or relate. Similar phenomena also occur in the human child. Long before the child can (correctly) speak, it has already gained untold impressions or experiences that are deeply engraved in its (implicit) memory and that automatically determine its actions.

Based on *circumstantial evidence*, I understood Bea's sensitivities and behaviour as post-traumatic reactions and/or as insecure attachment of the avoidant type. By way of overview and to help her see the forest for the trees, I offered constructs reasonably early on, which were vague but later, based on increasingly precise information and memories, referred to her father's impact. There were many indications that he was very volatile and unpredictable. He had problems with temper or emotion regulation, displayed alcohol abuse and transgressive behaviour, and possibly traumatised and terrorised his surroundings without being aware of much harm.

Especially when the problems seem to have existed for as long as the patient in question can remember, early constructions can help focus attention on specific unconscious formations. The initial hypothesis can be substantiated and clarified depending on the narrative or transference material within the therapeutic space. In Bea's case, this was amply the case. She has been in weekly psychotherapy with me for about two years (including a pregnancy break of several months). By positioning her sensitivities, hypervigilance, and distrust better, she has become more intimate with and emotionally close to her partner during that time. She can and sometimes dares to surrender and let go enough to enjoy it. She does retain some sensitivities or allergies from her father, but, by identifying the allergen in time, overly disastrous/severe (over)reactions are quietly avoided.

## Jessy—Something Wild

The patient is a younger-looking 30-something who was referred from a PWGH for inpatient psychotherapy. She had been hospitalised there several times following a severe alcohol intoxication and she complained of emotional volatility and instability.

Jessy is the elder of two daughters. The mother is educated and is described as a powerful, emotionally aware woman. On the other hand, she is said to be not very understanding. In reality, in Jessy's mind, she gets too close, verging on controlling and sometimes getting on her nerves. 'I have to keep her at bay.' As for her father, she had to perform well and conform to his ideal image. Thus, she was required to study classical humanities (Latin) and felt 'forced' into studies that were not her choice. She felt a bit trapped in a golden cage at home. Materially, she had everything she wanted, but she experienced no freedom and could not be exactly herself. There were many conflicts during puberty, especially with her father: 'I did the opposite'.

Jessy would have been a cheerful and energetic toddler but was a misfit from childhood. She clashed about clothes, her appearance in general, and going out. She felt like a 'showpiece'. From an early age, she sought to connect with older men. She tried to act 'big' but, owing to excessive docility, ended up suffering many abuses, including drug use and gang bang-like situations.

She has had a turbulent lifestyle for years, with volatile relationships and a hectic nightlife dominated by sex, drugs, and rock and roll. She feels adrift, unhinged. There is, at times, profuse alcohol abuse including binge drinking, resulting in blackouts. She has been running a dance bar for years. On the one hand, she feels like a kind of queen of the night, but soberly, chaos trumps all. All feeling is evacuated mainly in polytoxicomanic substance abuse and party intoxication. She seems empty-headed, *something wild*.

Jessy spent (only) about six months in inpatient psychotherapy. She experienced the regularity, safety, and structure of ward life as beneficial. A few times, things still went wrong at weekends, but she was able to analyse such incidents well afterwards and draw appropriate conclusions. She recognised that she had pushed her parents away, was rebellious, and wanted to be big and independent but was not. Her partner choices were symptomatic, bearing witness to the need for parental figures and, at the same time, resisting them. They were a form of being naughty with the punishment already baked in.

She was bright and streetwise but had very limited reflective or mentalising abilities. Just by being in our treatment environment and participating in various group activities, where emotional expression and communication are central, a world seemed to open up for her.

Also, considering the imperatives of her case, she was reluctantly (because, in her view, prematurely) discharged. Overlapping with a final phase in day therapy, she started weekly psychotherapy. Meanwhile, we are several years on. She still comes to me monthly for psychiatric and psychoanalytic process counselling. She is employed and lives in a 'happy cottage' together with her partner and their two young children.

### Heidi—Eight-Armed Holding

This 50-something woman was referred from a PWGH service where she had been hospitalised for the second time after a suicide attempt. In the first words of the introductory interview, she calls her life a mess. 'At the age of fourteen, I was sexually abused by my older brothers.' She says she has nothing left to live for.

Heidi is the third in a family of six children. Her sister committed suicide a long time ago because she was also a victim of sexual abuse. For the patient, this dragged on for several years, while the parents knew nothing about it and did not believe it when the daughters only very recently tried to discuss it: 'We are all liars, so to speak'.

Heidi married at 20 after a brief courtship 'to get away from home'. Her partner was brutal, verbally aggressive, and demeaning. Because of her sexual aversion, she was repeatedly raped within the marriage. In recent years, the couple lived 'like brother and sister'. They divorced about two years ago. An adult son sided with her wealthier ex, and she has no contact with him anymore. She does have a dog who means a lot to her emotionally. He is loyal and understands her without words. She also has good contact with one of her elder brothers and sister-in-law. He is a primitive man of few words but jumps in practically and helps her, and she feels believed and understood by him.

Heidi barely has any contact with her parents. She says she has no bond with them: 'They are like strangers'. The father is a professional soldier and described as authoritarian: he shouts and rants; his will is law, and everything has to be done his way. The mother is a calmer follower who is (also) afraid of the father. She is said to be sweet and understanding, yet has 'loose hands'.

Heidi has been scared, quiet, distrustful, a loner, and emotionally closed since childhood. The sexual abuse has left her with an aversion to sex and intimacy. She has always hidden everything from everyone, and the 'ulcer' only erupted a year ago.

Heidi had been in clinical psychotherapy with us for about a year. Apart from individual conversations here and there, she never dared to tell any more of her story. She was gagged and silenced to such an extent that hardly a word passed her lips. She remained majorly depressed and suicidal. She almost always spent the weekends (which are generally intended to maintain or develop contact with the natural environment) with us in the hospital.

While she was still hospitalised, we had her start outpatient psychotherapy close to home. Once some safety and trust had grown there, we organised psychiatric help at home provided by a satellite team from a so-called eight-armed psychiatric hospital in her neighbourhood.

It is reported that, three years later, she is now in and out of day treatment, still being cared for in their 'domain', under their various wings, and combining this with voluntary work. While many will perceive this as mere care, it rather concerns a recovery-oriented approach with a development assistance factor, which, as always, can only bear some fruit in the long run.

### Fanny—Body Language

Fanny is a 20-something referred for admission by her GP.

> I don't need to be there. There is no point in me being alive. I can't push these feelings away. I've always felt a bit like this. I already had problems at school, and now I'm being bullied at work. The whole group has turned against me. It's mainly to do with a jealous female colleague.

Or more: 'I have a weird head. I analyse everything from every possible point of view. I feel lonely'.

Fanny is the third of four children. She was the youngest for a long time. She didn't want this to change, as she felt comfortable with this status. She remembers a lot of hostile feelings from when she was ten, when her mother was pregnant with her younger sister. At birth, this was completely reversed. 'It was *my* daughter.' She devoted herself entirely to this little sister and cared for her constantly. 'The only thing I didn't do was get up at night.'

The father is a blue-collar worker. She describes him as a humorous man who laughs a lot. On the other hand, he is always ready to protect her. She has a good relationship with him and likes to feel seen. He is a 'correct' man who helps a lot in the household. The mother is said to be very caring and makes sure everything is in order. She is also immediately aware of everything. 'You can't hide anything from her.' She struggled many times herself. For instance, she went through severe depression before Fanny's birth as part of mourning the loss of *her* mother.

Fanny was a child who laughed a lot. Yet she was also scared and insecure. She had little self-confidence. Around the age of ten, she felt increasingly lonely and misunderstood. She then sought and found a lot of support from her dog. She felt lost. She remembers well how much she liked being allowed to sleep in her parents' room when her younger sister was away.

Fanny has always been very well-behaved and would never break the rules. She also has difficulty speaking. She can only answer direct questions. She is full of sadness and anger but can hardly express these feelings. From puberty onwards, she has sometimes scratched herself. She also developed a so-called tic disorder, for which she is under treatment by a neurologist. She takes a lot of medication for this, which, however, does not seem to help.

She makes involuntary movements with her head and body. 'Like trying to shake something off.' Sometimes, there are epileptiform seizures, in which, however, she does not lose consciousness. She had a job she enjoyed, but it was not without risk. Because of her symptoms, she has lost her job, and that is very painful.

In psychosomatic symptoms, 'unbound' and/or unmentioned contents exert a disturbing effect on mental and physical functioning in a raw and 'mute' manner. In conversion disorders, it is as if the body is speaking instead. The complaints or symptoms 'want to say something' that the patient is unaware of and/or that cannot be expressed in words.

Probably much less frequently than in general hospitals, such problems also occur in psychiatric hospitals. Blepharospasm, stuttering, semi-lateral neurological (dropout) symptoms, and various complaints of pain are then the proverbial tip of the iceberg. Invariably, an approach focusing on underlying psychodynamics or mental processes is enough to melt away such surface symptoms.

In Fanny's case, the nature or cause of her problem was not superficial. Searching and investigating were needed to get to the heart of the matter. She said: 'There is something, but I don't know what!' As she told her story, it turned out that, while she had received a lot of loving care and attention, she had not learned to speak the language of feelings precisely. On closer inspection, the 'smiley face' turned out to be the façade of a false self she had put up to be her depressed mother's sunshine.

*Sunny side up*—there were negative feelings that never saw the light of day. These were primarily impulses of anger and hatred towards her younger sister and mother, whom she took turns blaming for a loss of loving attention. They had accumulated to the point where the proverbial bucket had become full, and she could only shake off these aggressive feelings. Her cheerful appearance, then, contrasted with her severe and sometimes even downright alarming symptoms. Consequently, as she was no longer allowed to do the work she loved so much, she felt punished for the angry side of her nature.

Only thanks to, and in the course of, clinical psychotherapy did her emotional world unfold. For her, it was a liberation and a relief. The mask of the eternal smile disappeared, and she became more assertive in her relationship with her partner and at work.

## Gerda—Full of Silent Exclamation Marks

Gerda is in her early 20s and was hospitalised because of her suicidal thoughts and plans. By then, she had already been through three admissions of several months each and has also been in outpatient psychotherapy with various psychologists for many years. Immediately, she relates that she was sexually abused twice when she was still in primary school by an adolescent neighbour. He tricked and outsmarted her, cornered her, and sexually molested her in many ways while making death threats. Because he and her parents were friends, things remain covered up to this day. Even Gerda's younger siblings only know that 'something' allegedly happened at a summer camp.

Immediately after the 'facts', Gerda took a shower for hours in an attempt to cleanse herself. She then pushed everything away for years. She tried to be 'normal' and 'get along' with others, but, inside, she felt constantly anxious, distrustful, hurt, and abandoned. As a formality, she (like her peers) had a single relationship with a boy by whom she, once again, 'let herself be done'.

With regard to her childhood, Gerda describes herself as a rather gloomy child who never felt happy but was always an outcast. She saw only faults. Her parents often made her feel 'under pressure', both intellectually and emotionally. Her father she describes as a somewhat compulsive and perfectionist man who has to be able to predict and control everything in detail. He is also said to be somewhat on the rational side and has difficulty talking about feelings. Moreover, he used to have an alcohol problem. Under the influence, he 'blew his fuse' and could be pretty aggressive and short-tempered, so she would often come home thinking, 'How will Dad be today?'

Her mother is a rather anxious and hypersensitive woman who cannot take much. She experiences the relationship between her parents as somewhat cold, businesslike, and distant. Not much warmth or pleasure can be detected in them. In a way, she also finds both her parents a bit scared and weak. They try to avoid problems and conflicts. They both lack clout. For instance, Gerda recounts that she has commonly been the target of sexually transgressive/inappropriate comments made by her grandfather. She feels she is subjected to a humiliating and degrading kind of 'meat inspection' by him at those times. Note that this also happens in the presence of both her parents, who do not protect her in any way.

Because of her severe depression, with suicidal tendencies and self-harming behaviour, Gerda was in inpatient psychotherapy with us for many years. Periods of full (24-hour) hospitalisation alternated with periods of day treatment. Time and again, there is a flight forward into healing, but, to her discouragement and despair, she is also constantly overtaken by her own shadow.

She has a somewhat avoidant insecure attachment, keeping herself good, well-behaved, and robust so as not to burden her parents, and a strict and demanding conscience as characteristics she already has from before the trauma. She constantly tries to earn good marks. Meanwhile, she anxiously and compulsively keeps hidden post-traumatic re-experiences, flashbacks, and physical sensations, as well as a lot of anger, desire for revenge, pain, and grief.

She can hardly make these feelings manifest, show, or express them. Instead, she mindlessly drains them in the form of injuries that can be read as fleshly exclamation marks: 'Sometimes I would like to shout it all loudly from the rooftops'. To her great anger, the trauma has a lasting impact on all her psychosexual and psychosocial functioning. She can only get rid of the negative feelings by cutting into her flesh.

Throughout treatment, there was indeed very persistent self-mutilation that turned her genital area into an invisible battlefield. Despite all kinds of protective and safeguarding measures, she ended up in emergency rooms for this with clockwork regularity. Self-harm was, then, the less disastrous choice than suicide. It was 'carving not to die'.

It was also as if she wanted to cut out the rotten bits from an apple or the nauseating bits from a film. Not only can Gerda not forgive herself for her docility and compliant behaviour towards the boy next door, but she also knows she was not supposed to go with him. She allowed herself to be fooled—against her better judgement. She torments/punishes herself for her docility and 'collaboration' by ruthlessly mutilating herself.

As is well known, in play, the child actively tries to master and process experiences they have passively undergone. A child's play is an actual activity involving the symbolic use of various objects. Such passive–active reversal can make the child feel like a criminal monster when they are living objects (e.g., animals or other children). For example, Gerda played sexual games with boys despite not liking this at all. At that point, she felt like a perpetrator rather than a victim.

Even in young adulthood, there was sporadic acting-out where she had sex in brutal to violent ways, 'as if the devil was involved'. On one occasion, she said she deserved neither more nor less than the 'death penalty' for such things.

Gerda's treatment was a matter of sustained intensive care, support, attunement, and empathy, but also of precise surgery. It takes patient, precise work to separate healthy from diseased tissue and own from post-traumatic sexual experiences.

Gerda understands that her (dead) flesh is the opposite of a social, communicative, and erogenous body. And that changing this is necessary to escape the simultaneously pathetic and soulless existence of a zombie. We will probably be busy for quite some time with this kind of work, in the form of now twice-weekly outpatient psychotherapy.

## Sylvain—the (Be)Coming Man

This adolescent young man was hospitalised at the insistence of his father, a highly successful entrepreneur and businessman who has been in treatment for bipolar disorder for years and is functioning well and stable in all areas, thanks in part to taking lithium as a mood stabiliser. His first words: 'After I was born, my mother had postnatal depression. She allegedly developed schizophrenia and has been in a psychiatric institution continuously ever since'.

For the first two years of his life, Sylvain was with his paternal and maternal grandparents alternately. The former were from the upper middle class. They pampered and spoilt him very much. The other grandparents were a lot stricter and more restrictive. His father was not at home much owing to his busy professional activities. He met a new partner, and this woman 'emotionally adopted' Sylvain—fortunately, because Sylvain said he needed stability. He was scared, insecure, and hurt by all that was said about his mother. The stepmother may have cared for him, but she feared he would become like his mother. In the limited contact Sylvain had with his (biological) mother, he was very much at ease.

When he was in primary school, Sylvain was already very anxious and insecure. He felt awkward and stupid, constantly seeking attention and love from everyone by posturing and 'acting silly'. During secondary school, he gradually dropped classical humanities and switched to an apprenticeship in restoration. He has attention problems and, by his admission, is always dreaming. The trigger for admission was an anger outburst under the influence of alcohol. He hurled all kinds of reproaches and accusations at his father and wanted to slash the tyres of his car. Furthermore, Sylvain felt jealous of everyone and was so furious he was going to kill his mother.

Sylvain underwent about six months of inpatient psychotherapy. During this stay, he mainly dealt with deep feelings of abandonment. Sometimes he would fly into a primitive rage where he would lose his mind, as it were, and 'kick the crap' out of everyone. Afterwards, he felt very guilty and ashamed. It certainly did not fit into the well-educated picture he had to (and also wanted to) fit into for his father. His mother's psychiatric disorder (and accompanying emotional unavailability) had left Sylvain with a kind of narcissistic hurt. She was like a stain on his identity and instilled in him the fear that, sooner or later, he, too, would become psychotic.

Residential treatment made a big difference, especially regarding basic safety and building/restoring a positive sense of self. Thus, he has since been in outpatient counselling for more than a decade. Periods of weekly psychotherapy alternate with periods of low-frequency contact, but the line has always remained open, and he manages to maintain a relationship of trust to this day.

Sylvain has had steady work for many years, bought his flat with his father's financial help, and has a stable relationship with a woman who is sufficiently realistic and solid to care for her boyfriend. In fact, he mostly still struggles with more Oedipal themes. For instance, he wants to be as big and important as his father. Now and then, professional ambitions flare up that he simultaneously knows (and is reminded by those around him) are too high for his true abilities.

He also occasionally loses himself in the nightlife scene, trying to be 'the big guy' by buying drinks he can't afford, among other things. Finally, he occasionally goes off the rails and visits a brothel or flirts with different women on social media. He is aware that he does this to boost his phallic sense of self, but it is sometimes even stronger than himself. He tightens the bow a little whenever he encounters such 'symptoms'. He intensifies his psychotherapy appointments for a while until a new knot is untangled or a new cliff can be sidestepped without too much trouble.

## Hugo—Tom and Jerry

Hugo is a 50-something working as a salesman. He presents himself with his head bowed and between his shoulders and adopts a remarkably submissive attitude in contact. He has been on the mend for several years from depressive symptoms, for which he was briefly hospitalised at a PWGH service several times. The last time, he was treated with electroconvulsive therapy, but this had no result. He says he sleeps badly because of problems at work. The clients keep getting more complex and more demanding. He feels powerless and abused.

Conflicts arise increasingly, with legal proceedings even being initiated. It is all very stressful and 'driving me *crazy*'. He adds: 'I've been beaten all my life!' There is also a 'peeing problem'. He feels an urge to urinate, but 'nothing comes out'. So he goes to the toilet countless times a day and is constantly afraid he won't be able to hold it in. Yet, each time, it turns out to be a 'false alarm'.

Hugo is the eldest of three in a farming family. His mother died several years before. He describes her as a hard worker. She was very fond of order and cleanliness but otherwise hot-tempered and aggressive. She occasionally clipped him around the ear for no reason or to an out-of-proportion degree. This last happened when he was already in his early 20s. He felt mistreated by her and experienced a lot of feelings of powerlessness and injustice. From childhood, Hugo was subdued and embarrassed. As a result, he was also bullied and excluded at school. 'It left me with a feeling of inferiority that I never got rid of.' He harboured a lot of resentment towards his mother. She is said to have once chased him with a butcher's knife. 'I don't know what a mother is.' His father has also died and is described as having been a calm, quiet man who did not dare contradict Mother, his wife. The father and son understood each other without words.

Hugo spent a long time in the army after secondary school on the advice of his father ('steady work!') and made some career progress there. He never liked his job there, clashing all the time with superiors who were very strict and to whom he could not speak. He says he is happily married to a strong woman who works in the care sector and 'takes charge'. The now-grown-up children are coping and seem to have found their way in life. However, Hugo has since concluded that he wanted to do things differently to his mother, educationally. He set few boundaries, exercised little authority, and, on closer inspection, spoilt his children. As a result, they show him little gratitude or respect, even though he has already done and paid for all sorts of things for them.

Hugo underwent an episode of clinical psychotherapy for about three months. There, he gained (mainly cognitive) insight into the origins of his weak phallic sense of self and his aggression inhibition, especially against (maternal) superiors. He felt castrated, identified with the father, and was more or less continuously depressed or upset, with all the bladder and urinary problems that this entailed.

Since his admission, he has been coming for outpatient consultations for psychiatric (he takes a maintenance dose of antidepressants) and psycho-analytic process counselling for about a decade now. On my referral, he was in weekly psychotherapy for two periods of several years. In this, we note that, each time, he clashes with psychodynamics in variations on the theme. The resistance/repression is enormous. We have already had numerous sessions where convincing evidence and confirmation of the mentioned hypotheses have been found, based on dream material and free association. Nevertheless, the subsequent conversation reveals that he is ignorant of his inner self, and the wheel must be reinvented repeatedly.

On his initiative, he occasionally visits more or less alternative healers. On two occasions, he has consulted a fellow psychiatrist who gives different advice, pharmacologically and psychotherapeutically. He then submits the second/third opinion to me with an open face and observes how I react to such disobedience/sniping.

In other words, the cat-and-mouse game with his mother has also gradually emerged in the transference. Through our being able to discuss it in live encounters and interaction, the initial rational realisation makes way for a more felt and lived-through one. Recent quote: 'I appreciate that you never exactly blame me for my visits to other therapists!' The fact that someone can be traitor to their therapist and still not be punished or rejected for it is not in line with his deeply held beliefs.

## Godfrey—a Flemish Lion

Godfrey is in his late 40s and was referred from a PWGH service, where he has already been hospitalised several times because of serious suicide attempts. One of his daughters filed a complaint against him for incest. He was arrested by the police and spent a short time in custody but was finally found not guilty in court.

However, the whole thing caused him to lose everything in one fell swoop. He lost his job, his wife initiated divorce proceedings, and the children were kept away from him. On admission, he is a broken man. He feels very much wronged. It turns out he has always been an ardent Flemish fighter. He has been affiliated with various far-right and Flemish-nationalist associations for many years and, in every community conflict, he goes to stand on the barricades or comes to blows with the police and other activists. Consequently, he feels he has been targeted by Belgian state security.

Godfrey was the eldest in a family of 11 children. Father was himself a fanatical Flemish nationalist. He served a prison sentence for collaboration after the Second World War. He suffered from alcoholism, but Godfried calls him 'a real comrade'. His mother was extremely obese. He tells all sorts of anecdotes full of obscene to abject details about her menstruation, shameless nudity, and public masturbation. He was once almost crushed by her because she had fallen on him half-dressed. He is full of disgust, fear, and anger towards his mother, whom he cannot help but call 'a bitch'.

Partly owing to his father's imprisonment, Godfrey had to work hard from an early age to help support the family. His childhood was all about fighting and hard labour. With his wife, it was love at first sight. He often tells and repeats how she came cycling by 'like a gift from heaven', and he immediately thought, 'That will be the mother of my children!' They have been happily married for over 20 years, in his opinion, and have four children. Even though they have since divorced and she wants nothing to do with him, he loves her 'dearly'.

Godfrey always did a lot of hard, heavy, and dangerous work 'for my wife and my family'. He was very politically driven and committed to far-right Flemish nationalism. He is uneducated but follows national and international politics through the press and media. His discourse is coherent. He is convinced of his rightness and determined to hold combative views on anything and everything.

On closer inspection, he holds pretty sophisticated and nuanced views, but his core values are the traditional family, law and order, devout Catholicism, and classical gender roles and relationships. He went as far as to fight for them in neighbouring foreign countries, especially against socialists, libertines, and, more generally, various forms of (in his view) social degradation. 'Perhaps I put too much time and energy into it and thus neglected my wife and children without knowing it or wanting to?'

Indeed, Godfrey has wondered countless times what could have possessed his daughter to accuse him of such an outrage. Perhaps he was too strict? Too conservative in his views? Too absent, because he was away from home owing to a lot of work, not to mention his relentless political struggles on literal and figurative barricades, at home and abroad?

He was in inpatient psychotherapy for about two years, the second half of it in day treatment.

He was severely depressed for a long time and also attempted suicide while in hospital. He gradually started to feel safer and more at home with us, was able to tell his story, and, in doing so, made himself small and vulnerable. Whereas initially he enveloped himself in a hypermasculine and, at the same time, somewhat misogynistic attitude and views, a considerable softening occurred. He became more aware of his beliefs' emotional and filial roots, which caused him to move politically towards the middle.

Living in the deprived suburb of a provincial town, he saw the population moving towards an increasingly exotic multiculturality. In social services, where he went to do some voluntary work, he remained silent when surrounded by leftist progressive utterances and ideas. This was mainly owing to the development of mental and integrative processes, where black-and-white thinking had given way to more moderation and nuance. Towards the end, he combined day therapy with volunteering at a social centre.

Of great therapeutic importance was the following: at the heart of the ward is an art studio. It is a kind of heterotopia or sanctuary where patients can play under the inspiring and animating guidance of an artist who has no therapeutic training and does not comment (and certainly not psychologically) on their production. This was a revelation for Godfrey—a musical register he could enjoy to the full.

Since then, he has been coming for monthly sessions for about 15 years. Occasionally, there are still waves of outrage in response to news events or social changes in his immediate surroundings. He often, pertinently, reads trifles as surface manifestations of implicit ideological tendencies that pass most of us entirely by. For him, I am a port of call and point of contact where he can find an understanding ear in an atmosphere of positive acceptance. He has been 'using' me all these years as a kind of developmental object based on which his mentalising and integrative capacity continues to grow steadily.

When some re-establishment of contact with three of his children came gradually, he wore the textile bracelet given to him by one of his daughters for months (until it wore out)—a piece of jewellery that would have been unthinkable for him to wear in his earlier, hypermasculine days. He had to watch sorrowfully as one son joined the Indignado movement, and another began a relationship with a sub-Saharan African.

Occasionally, there is still some depressive relapse or some paranoid-tinged fears and experiences. He maintains a stable positive transference expressed by many signs of gratitude and great confidence. He adheres to our monthly contacts, which are quite an emotional boost for him in sometimes magical ways.

Recent mental health developments involving socialisation of care recently made it possible to set up some home counselling. It is meant to bring him more out of passivity and isolation and alleviate some of his social and economic poverty. I feared it would be a delicate exercise for the counsellors. Wouldn't he perceive their home visit as interference and the anxious attention as somewhat unwanted surveillance and control?

To my pleasant surprise, none of this was the case at all. He opened the door and his heart to the young female social workers who came to his place. However, he kept all of the too-intimate and painful details of his history to himself. 'With my dirty laundry, I can get more than enough here!'

## Richard—Burning Love

Behold Richard's first words during our introductory interview:

> When I was two years old, my mother crashed. She crashed into a petrol station and was burnt alive. My father processed this with difficulty. He was silent about it. So, everything was buried along with my mother. I have no memories of my mother or a picture of her. After this tragedy, my father got into a quarrel with the grandmother on my mother's side, as well as with the rest of her family. As a result, I no longer have any contact with them. I had to go to them from the justice of the peace, but my father prevented this. Thus, my grandmother also (!) dropped me. I missed something all my life: motherly love and affection.

Richard is the youngest of four. The other children also have manifest mental health problems. The eldest brother, for instance, is on the wrong path in the form of drug abuse and petty crime. Both sisters are in conflict with anyone and everyone. He used to be a 'living doll' to them. They cuddled and patronised him.

The father is described as rigid and insensitive and prefers to keep away from his children as much as possible. He has since remarried a stepmother Richard describes as a lovely woman who does her utmost. Richard was with the youth movement from childhood and spent two months every summer with his paternal grandmother. He sought and found support from friends and did his best to be liked. He has never been carefree or really himself. He is sweet towards everyone, does all he is asked, and puts on a mask everywhere to feel important. 'I close up when the relationship gets too intense, too intimate, too real', because he feels inferior to everyone.

He consumed a lot of alcohol and drugs during his adolescence and also spent some time in a gang. 'I have a small heart, but I play the tough one.' 'Brave' is written in shaky letters on his T-shirt. It often happens that words on clothing speak volumes. In this case, even in two languages (in Dutch 'brave' means well-behaved). Richard attended general secondary school and worked in a factory for several years. He describes his boss as a dirty bastard who constantly singles him out and hounds him. He does not have much contact there because he does not connect with colleagues.

Richard had been in clinical psychotherapy for just under a year. Despite his macho and somewhat heavy-metal-like appearance, he quickly won the hearts of fellow patients and the team. Consequently, he was lovely, affectionate, and, as it is called, 'eager to please' in contact. He visibly enjoyed the emotional care and attention that are so central and eagerly participated in all activities and therapies.

Two things played a prominent role in his significant progress there. First, there was a positive 'click' with me as a psychiatrist. Although negative father transference was among the expectations, there was little of this. Above all, a colossal father hunger was satisfied by some of the non-specific characteristics of any therapeutic relationship—empathy, calm firmness, and, last but not least, positive acceptance.

Furthermore, there was persistent self-harm, with him burning both forearms with a lighter, sometimes almost daily, for months. When we understood this, again and again, as a combination of identification with, and fusional longings for, his deceased mother, many split-off and unintegrated feelings of abandonment, depression, and anger emerged and were raised.

Unprocessed grief and loss, as well as pent-up anger towards the father, were discussed at length. Defusing this explosive stopped the self-mutilating behaviour. Dreams reflected how he cherished the scars of his burns as a relic or a souvenir.

After his admission, he started (and has since completed) a training programme as an educator. He started working with behaviourally disturbed adolescents. He still came for only low-frequency outpatient consultations because, from the peace of mind he had acquired, it seemed that the suffering was over. For a few years afterwards, I systematically received a Christmas card with many thanks and best wishes. Now and then, he accompanies young people who are hospitalised or treated in our hospital.

### Gregory—Il Papa Che Non Si Trova

His GP referred this 30-something tour guide after treatment with various antidepressants and three short admissions to a psychiatric hospital in his area had produced a slight improvement. He says he feels bad in his skin and immediately and spontaneously relates this to his childhood and upbringing in which he felt accepted nowhere and was often bullied and excluded.

His father is a teacher. He used to have a severe alcohol addiction but is said to have been 'clean' for many years. According to the patient, he was a good, hardworking, and driven person. He was also popular and liked everywhere, and 'we allegedly made problems that were not there'. Meanwhile, indoors and under the influence of alcohol, there were many quarrels, with shouting and ranting but also physical violence, where the mother and children had to flee to their grandmother and aunt. 'I never had a father figure.' This misery was fearfully and convulsively kept hidden, as the mother wanted to keep up appearances at all costs.

By his own account, the patient put on a mask, which was also expected of him in an unspoken way by his mother. The latter is described as a strong woman who wants the best for her children. Only gradually is more anger expressed towards her because of her covering up ('curtains down') and hypocrisy. An older brother still lives at home, also has problems with alcohol abuse, and is still a virgin and single at the time.

As a toddler, Gregory was cheerful and good-natured. He mainly played with girls and suffered quite a bit of bullying as a result. He had few friends in primary school and did not participate in sports and games. He was sent to a boarding school to learn hospitality management, where he turned out to be a bit of a posing rooster who showed negative attention-seeking behaviour but did not feel at home at all.

By his admission, Gregory leads a volatile and irregular, vagrant existence. He has never had a steady partner and repeatedly falls for the 'wrong' men. Either they are promiscuous and only eager for homosexual contact, or they are straight and neither able nor willing to reciprocate his (need for) affection. 'Maybe I am too perfectionist or too demanding?'

Gregory began with a six-month admission to inpatient psychotherapy. He was a 'rebel without a cause' almost all the time there. He went into battle with all the therapists, systematically challenging rules and boundaries, rebelling against even the slightest perceived forms of authority, and complaining about the lack of care and commitment on the part of the team.

He also takes a hard line against what he calls the psychoanalytic working principles of the department, against the way patients are treated, against the 'system' of exit and visitation. Whereas these attacks and criticisms are initially directed at the department's heads, he gradually aims his arrows more and more definitely at me as the departmental psychiatrist in charge of policy. Accusations of perceived lack of understanding, heartlessness, a too-harsh hand, or too authoritarian treatment are not uncommon.

Initially, we let him calm down and tried to maintain a calm and sustained empathic mindset in the face of his destructive attacks. We invited him to tell his story and recount his history in all sorts of ways so that, even without our transference cues, he began to notice parallels in his experience and make the necessary connections himself, not least with all kinds of negative experiences and trials with his father in the past.

When this storm of negative feelings had sufficiently subsided, the conversations became more about his homosexual orientation. He could and dared to assume it more and began to discuss his amorous quests and mishaps in more intimate detail. When he started to get some overview of his life and the patterns that were repeating themselves, we switched to weekly outpatient psychotherapy.

Except for a few breaks during which he comes monthly or somewhat more irregularly, he has had a weekly face-to-face session for about a decade. During this period, we have been able to take a closer look at his love life. He was repeatedly drawn into unrequited infatuations with rugged and tough men who were married but doubted their heterosexual orientation. He yearned for their love and physical expressions of love but lost out again and again, rejected because they ultimately chose their families.

We all have only one father and mother and only one period of life in which we can have their extraordinary love. Where or with whom else but them can this *spring* (necessary for our emotional well-being) be found? And, when we think we do see it in someone, it turns out that the man in question is not gay but straight! Or a heterosexual who doubts or is in turmoil about his homosexual feelings. Or a straight man who is married and the father of children, so he can't or won't ever really choose Gregory.

Gregory also explored his pickiness. He discovered that he was chasing a kind of dream image of a virile guy who could both support and hold him and who would treat him with the tenderness and affection he so sorely missed. He cruised parks and petrol stations in search of contacts who satisfied him only to a minimal extent. A pivotal moment in his psychotherapy was a dream in which he stood in his mother's shoes, archetypically leaning against a tough guy with one leg bent and raised.

We had talked about his father hunger many times in variations on the theme. Still, the negative Oedipal constellation of identification with the mother and craving for the father was thus conclusively proven. At the same time, the realisation germinated that finding the ideal partner was utterly impossible, and he would have to make do with *the next best thing* anyway.

Until then, with every budding relationship, he had kept the door ajar for a different and better partner that might still cross his path. He became more open to, and less critical of, potential love partners. He also discovered what was behind his so-called 'reservedness': the fear of committing to a man. Love necessarily implies a dependency where he feels at the mercy of the other person's power. He is terrified of defencelessness and the vulnerability this entails.

At some point, the repetition, if not inevitable certainty, of difficulties became sufficiently clear to him. Although it might have looked obvious to an outsider, for Gregory, it created a liberating Eureka moment. Since then, he has been unable to discuss his dating adventures without the necessary distance and humour. He manages to be respected when he feels his feelings are being played with. Although he remains hopeful of finding the True One, he can open up more and enjoy less promising encounters and contacts.

Other themes that often came up in his work situation were abandonment, anger, and rebellion. In the tourism industry, an indestructible toothpaste smile is a must. Extraordinary anger appeared to be hidden behind the friendly and cheerful façade he had to present. At the same time, internally, he was weighed down by unbearable feelings because he was misunderstood and not seen by anyone. Sometimes, he felt like bursting out and slapping the honoured customer around the face!

He also gradually started looking at the broader picture. While he long viewed his father as the culprit and his mother as the victim of his drinking, a more nuanced picture of the situation emerged. How overbearing his mother was, how she was focused on 'keeping up appearances', how degrading and 'castrating' she could be sometimes when she raged against his father, and how 'good' his father was when he had not been drinking.

Despite his close relationship and identification with his mother, he comes into contact with a factor of parentification. Didn't both sons have to fill a vacancy willy-nilly? Did they each, in their way, not marry their mother above all else? Were they not able or allowed to detach themselves sufficiently from home?

Indeed, according to Gregory, the older brother is also stuck in a lopsided triangle. He still lives at home, has a huge drinking problem, and has had only a few relationships that never last very long; he constantly protects his mother and can sometimes lash out at his father, only to be calm again for a while. Gregory was glad that, (only) on the occasion of his admission to our home, he had moved out and thus had been able to escape the (he said jokingly: Bermuda) triangle a lot better.

## Lia—Done with Settling

Lia is a coquettish 50-year-old woman who had been in outpatient therapy for several years when she was referred for inpatient psychotherapy. 'I have low self-esteem. I am miserable. I am afraid I will do something to myself.' She is a single, divorced mother. She has an adolescent son who has been in a relationship for several months. 'I have lost him.' Caring for her son has always kept her straight; now she fears 'falling into a big black hole'.

She married her first sweetheart, Herman, in her early 20s. In retrospect, they were both very young and naive. They independently ran a tavern and a discotheque, and, partly owing to the nightlife environment, her husband started drinking more and more, becoming more dominant at home and even physically aggressive. Lia soon met another man by whom she immediately became pregnant, so they started living together. He was an avid angler and left her for another woman after two years.

Then followed a long-term living-apart-together relationship with a much older man with whom she had a blinkered relationship. Within the relationship, he was stifling and controlling. Whenever she tried to break off the relationship, he started stalking her. She has been working in home care for the last few years after training as a nursing assistant. She does her job there with total dedication. She notes that her colleagues are much less strict about punctuality and workload. Somehow, all the difficult and dirty jobs are hers.

Lia is the third of six children. Her father passed away. He was a blue-collar worker but was on disability for most of his life because of back problems. She describes him as sickly but also as a very demanding, stubborn, and childish man with many quirks and whims. 'Everyone has to jump when he says.' Her mother was a kitchen help and a tough, strong woman. 'I wouldn't have been able to do what she managed: stay with father and care for six children.' On the other hand, she says she had nothing from her mother—no love, attention, or support.

Lia was scared, insecure, timid, quiet, and naive from childhood. After all, at home, there were always arguments, with her father shouting and ranting and threatening violence. There was never peace for long. Lia was never rebellious, never came out of the corner or stood up for herself. She always obediently did as she was asked. She hardly had any friends or girlfriends. She did go 'running/jogging' (*sic*) regularly, though. Even in recent years, she has been doing Zumba and fitness.

Lia was in clinical psychotherapy for about six months. When I saw her, a poet's verse came to mind: 'And ah, let the girls arrange their feathers. And smile'. So she has, and cultivates, something graceful, is always dressed very well, and seeks to people-please constantly.

At the same time, and paradoxically, she is also unremarkable. She is quiet and speaks quietly, follows her therapy programme obediently and docilely, and demands little attention or care. Rather, she is very gentle and sweet to everyone. It takes a long time before she starts expressing her own needs and anger because they are overlooked and met even less.

She becomes more aware along the way that she is servile to earn love. She is always slavishly submissive, trying to avoid any attack and appease possible aggressors. She has always been very focused on caring for her son. For a while, she was worried that he would develop homosexuality. Although he was often involved with girlfriends, she felt he indulged too much in women's affairs and made few moves on the romantic front.

Meanwhile, she was discharged several years ago. She is in weekly psychotherapy. With the medical adviser's permission, she trained as a pedicurist and started working independently. In this regard, she has introduced herself to a few GPs, rest and care homes, and even shoe shops.

Behind the attraction and rejection because of her last husband, she has been able to make a definite point. She now wants to continue as a single person for quite some time. She never misses an opportunity to correct men if something does not suit her. First and foremost, she wants to enjoy her newly conquered freedom and has no intention of letting it be taken away from her. And definitely not by the first person who tries to charm her with compliments and sweet words. Fortunately, I don't need that kind of affirmation anymore!

Her problems were relatively simple, and the psychotherapeutic process was mainly emancipatory, using awareness and increased empowerment. A psychodynamic approach is often effective, even in its basic form. Provided there are sustained receptivity and willingness to listen, the patient speaks for themself without fuss.

## Marianne—a French Revolution

Marianne is a 40-something teacher referred by her GP for inpatient psychotherapy.

> I've been at home for two years. It started with severe depression: crying and sadness all the time. I don't feel like doing anything. I was a bit burnt out because of my work. The split between my father and youngest brother, Jef, greatly affected me. Jef got divorced, and our father could neither accept nor stomach it. My son's transition to secondary school also did not go smoothly. He set the bar lower than me. I was worried that he would not get a good degree, but I am glad that he is not as perfectionist as I am. I worried a lot and felt myself sinking. I have been in treatment with a psychiatrist all along. He has tried all possible anti-depressants. In an attempt to return to work earlier this year, I had to give up after about three months.

Marianne is the eldest of three. Her father is an executive in the financial sector. He is very punctual and precise. Everything must always be in order, or he can't stand it. He is said to have suffered from depression himself. Her mother is an administrative clerk and she is pretty disciplined. She has a good disposition and is helpful, but the children must obey her without question.

From a young age, Marianne was energetic but also doubtful and insecure. She has difficulty making decisions and always goes to her mother for advice. She tends to underestimate herself and suffers a lot from exam anxiety and fear of failure. By her admission, this is owing to both parents' high demands and expectations of her, whether implicit or explicit. She always wanted to be top of the class and was heartbroken if even one test did not go well.

She is married to an 'exact' scientist who is an industry executive. She felt it was essential to find a partner who was more capable than her, which made her feel secure. They love each other, but there is little, arduous communication. Her husband is very closed-minded. He is rational and straightforward in his thinking. Emotional understanding is not his strong suit.

It is probably evident to the outsider that Marianne has been walking on eggshells all her life. She does her utmost to meet expectations and avoid comments or criticism. At the same time, she harbours a lot of anger and rebellion towards all those (in her eyes) in power around her. Emancipation starts with awareness. It is a necessary but insufficient condition. It is followed by a movement towards liberation and struggle for independence, ideally conducted verbally or at a (negotiating) table.

Marianne had only had an intake of about three months, enough to realise the pattern in which she had become stuck. Some three years of weekly out-patient psychotherapy followed, during which she fought her way free. She never missed an opportunity to connect the dots at work and in her family.

She was very combative and armed to the teeth and (not without pleasure) turned out to be a kitten to be handled with gloves.

It is a problem when resistance often comes more from the environment. Both her husband and father repeatedly emailed me with all kinds of complaints because of the (for them) unwelcome evolution. In the context of process counselling, I had three conversations with Marianne and her husband. It was clear from the last one that the balance of power had almost been reversed rather than corrected. In the meantime, her husband sat there looking very bedraggled and with his tail between his legs. Under the motto thesis, antithesis, and synthesis, the future will tell whether the pendulum can find the middle.

## Muriel—a Storm in a Glass of Water

This middle-aged woman had already had several short admissions to a PWGH service in the last year when she was referred for further and more in-depth psychotherapy. 'All my inner life is surfacing. The ulcer has erupted.' Muriel is chairwoman of a socio-cultural association. War broke out within this circle thanks to what was perceived as a scandal. Two married couples broke up as a result of a love affair. There is much turmoil around this issue, with supporters and opponents of this or that party. Consequently, there is a feud within the municipality where she lives.

Muriel finds herself in the eye of this storm, feeling responsible and compromised, which led her to resign because of accusations of bias. Although she knows she had nothing to do with the whole affair, she hardly dares to go outside out of shame. Apart from all this, she is happily married with two grown-up children who seem to be finding their way in life quite well.

Muriel is the eldest of six children from a farming family. Her mother died a year before. She is described as a sweet and gentle woman. 'She would care much less about all that.' Her father also died, much longer ago. He was a somewhat closed but socially minded and concerned man.

During the first conversation, it already comes up that a tragedy occurred during her childhood. A brother then turned to crime owing to an unfortunate coincidence. The whole village was in uproar then, and her family was gossiped about and disgraced. It was hard for her to deal with all that, but she took it all very much to heart and suffered a lot of guilt, even though—being a primary school child herself—she had done nothing wrong.

It was distressing for her that, in the wake of recent events, these facts from the past were brought up again and even thrown in her face by some. She, therefore, needs a place of refuge and help to get her mind off things.

On admission, Muriel was very anxious and depressed. She felt restless and hunted. Given her otherwise clear history and the fact that she had until recently led what she said was a happy and fruitful life, we understood her condition to be depressive adjustment disorder. The Gestalt of the whole current event chimed with that of the drama in her childhood and was like a trigger that caused unmentalised and disconnected (post-)traumatic contents to break through to the surface.

We let her tell her story extensively and repeatedly, connecting the here and now with back then. In this sense, our approach was very focused. However, this psychotherapeutic approach was offered within the emotionally caring, maternal environment of the ward.

Although she lived nearby, we kept her in full hospitalisation for the necessary period so that she could contemplate the current situation with sufficient distance and look back on the past. We let her enter daycare only once the emotional storm had subsided sufficiently. When her return to the village went without a hitch, and she had also been able to take up her membership and even presidency again, we switched to outpatient follow-up.

A bridge that looks solid and has often remained standing for a long time—despite the heavy traffic that has thundered over it day in, day out—can nevertheless suddenly collapse. It has to do with a highly exceptional but fatal kind of resonance phenomenon that spectacularly reveals a hidden defect. The constellation of scandals in the village community resonated with old situations that had embarrassed Muriel even then. Though her mind could well see the futility of the scandal in our modern times, it evoked intense and still undigested feelings 'as if it were yesterday'.

In contrast to the horizontal phenomenon of displacement, there are the vertical ones of fission and dissociation. Of course, these are only ideal-typical concepts because the naturalism of the clinic is always characterised by (put playfully) diagonal phenomena.

What is certain is that a whole complex of emotions and modes of reaction had been stored, virtually intact, beyond the reach of Muriel's conscious awareness all these years. It came to the fore with all its disruptive impact in response to a trigger that fitted like a key in the lock. The task was then to mentalise and articulate the undigested in order to let it 'sink in' enough to avoid further eruptions.

Now, a year later, there is no trace of psychological suffering. She no longer seeks real psychotherapy. She came for consultations, first monthly and then quarterly. In retrospect, the nightmare she had fallen into was reduced to an evil dream. The adultery that became public could be looked back on as a storm in a teacup. Or as the *fait divers* (trivial event) it had also become in a rural environment in the early 21st century.

## Nora—Almost Happy

Nora is a 20-something with a very delicate and fragile appearance and is referred by a neurologist with whom she is undergoing treatment for head and other pain symptoms. Her first words:

I am struggling with myself. I cough up everything from before. I find it hard to talk. I shut myself off completely. I see everything black, feel internally nervous, and can't eat or sleep. I feel alone, abandoned and a bit ashamed.

On enquiry, she also appears to have suicidal thoughts and plans.

Nora's parents divorced when she was eight years old. She caught her father with another woman and told her mother, which then the ball got rolling. Since then, her father has vanished with a vengeance, apart from a rare New Year or birthday card. She attaches great importance to truth and honesty but, on the other hand, lives with the fact that, 'by snitching on daddy', she played a decisive role in her parents' divorce.

Her father was a critical, hot-tempered figure who constantly criticised her. She did miss her father and kept hoping and waiting for any sign of life or love from him. Her mother is described as having a big mouth and a small heart. She can be very harsh, blunt, and hurtful. 'She is a real blabbermouth.' She never received much warmth or many hugs from her mother.

Since childhood, Nora has had various physical complaints. She had bladder and kidney problems, for which there were multiple hospitalisations. In recent years, there have also been a lot of health problems following road accidents in which she was hit by drunk drivers, resulting in a lot of fractures and painful residual complaints.

After the divorce, her mother started another relationship. This new partner sexually abused Nora on several occasions between the ages of 10 and 12. She did not tell her mother this until they broke up. Her mother was not bothered about this and, after this break-up, went to live abroad 'to start a new life'.

Nora was on her own then, having to continue running her mother's sandwich shop, but she was happy being looked after by her great-grandmother and her grandfather, both of whom she describes as 'her God' and admires immensely. The grandfather has since passed away, and she still misses him every day. She says she can hardly get over this loss. She is also terrified of losing her great-grandmother sooner or later.

So far, Nora has had two relationships with girls. She is somewhat tangled up in these but finds more understanding and gentleness in women, while she is distrustful and opposed to men.

Nora was in inpatient psychotherapy for about a year. Since then, she has been coming to consultations roughly monthly for about 20 years. The conversations have a psychodynamic slant. Nora herself returns to themes or topics that have been dealt with, or she picks out from the countless events of the past period those moments that seem meaningful for her problems.

In each conversation, she brings one or more formations of her unconscious: a dream, an emotional experience, or a course of action that is incomprehensible to herself. I make connections to the history of her feelings, and she produces free associations that substantiate, illustrate, or complement them.

She would love to come more and even opt for readmission, but she is so restricted financially that she and her steady friend have struggled to make ends meet every month for years. She needs more emotional care and support than I can offer her at this low frequency. She also says she would like to work on her psychotherapy 'more intensively'.

Neither parent ever provided attention or space for emotional expression or experience. It was straightforward work and carry on. With her great-grand-mother and grandfather, she did find the necessary tender loving care she had missed with her parents. Consequently, she is devoted to them and worships them like saints.

Two events scarred her mentally: first, her father's adultery. 'I saw Christine [her father's mistress] under my parents' bed for the first time.' Of course, she immediately understood what this meant and told her mother straight away. Her punishment for this truth-telling was cruel. Her father disappeared from the scene, and she has not seen him again. Truth versus lie and deception have remained sensitive issues for her. She has a nose for hypocrites and swindlers, who seem to surround her.

Another event that defined her life to the greatest extent was the sexual abuse by her mother's boyfriend. He was a prominent and obese figure who overwhelmed her not only mentally but also physically, almost crushing her. Threatened with death, she endured his sexual assaults for about two years, and it was only after her mother left him that she told her the facts.

Her mother believed her, but she did not receive much emotional support or understanding. She has been left with a complex post-traumatic stress disorder from this unpleasant period that is ingrained in her character. There is excessive vigilance. 'I have eyes in the back of my head.'

This is a blessing in specific circumstances, as she can see real dangers from a mile off, but it is also a curse. After all, she does not experience much peace and relaxation. Not only does she see things that others do not (yet) see, but she is also very suspicious of big-headed bosses she sees around her all the time. When she is confronted with certain traits from the perpetrator's Gestalt, this evokes raw and intense emotional reactions that completely unsettle her.

Nora had only a brief relationship with a boy until she broke it off because of his sexual pressuring. Otherwise, she remained a small but brave child, at home with her mother and grandparents for many years. She helped the former 'day and night' in the sandwich shop, and, as for the latter, she took care of them with almost religious devotion until they died, one after the other, with all the pain and mourning that entailed.

For the last ten years, she has been living with a steady girlfriend in a relationship based on care, gentleness, understanding, and satisfaction of deep oral needs and wants. Unfortunately, she has inherited very persistent head and neck pain, among other issues, from the various 'accidents' caused by 'arse-holes'. Apart from that, she has found peace and security in her relationship. 'If my body did not punish me so much, I would almost call myself happy.'

## Olga—Footloose

Olga is a flamboyant 30-something who tells her story with great poise, not mincing words.

> I was in a PWGH for several weeks and have already spent three months in an observation and treatment centre when I was fourteen. I start freaking out. I am fleeing. I was living in my car for the past two weeks. I love my boyfriend to death. Also, my little one. Also, his children. But the closer people get to me, the madder I get. I have to leave then. I need a 20-mile distance.

Olga's parents divorced when she was three years old. Her father had several sweethearts. Her mother was an alcoholic. Her mother then moved in with a neighbour, and this man immediately started sexually abusing and raping Olga. 'I had to jerk him off and suck him off.' This happened every morning and every night. Her mother knew about it, but she seemed like a pimp. She used Olga as a kind of shield. 'She put me on my stepfather's lap!' The man was not only abusive but also extremely violent. On several occasions, he wanted to kill her with his car. 'He was a supporter of Hitler.' He controlled her and constantly curtailed her freedom of movement.

From the age of 12, Olga made murder plans. She looked up the methods she could use in an encyclopaedia. She did, however, hesitate about whom she would eliminate first. Early in high school, she was placed in a closed institution by the juvenile court. She was unruly at school, ran away from home for three weeks, and wrote a letter to the Centre for Pupil Guidance, but this only got the court ball rolling. Her stepfather and mother ran up convictions, but the former haunts her. He has friends in the police and politics. She describes him as a man wholly outside and above the law. 'There is nothing to be done about it!'

Olga is a sensible woman. She has managed to get a degree despite everything. She has completed several higher vocational courses and has worked for several employers for long periods and to the satisfaction of all concerned. However, she has been using cannabis, cocaine, speed, and ecstasy for years. She is in a very intense relationship with her current partner. She is very greedy in her sexual activities, which she describes openly, completely shamelessly, and in full colour. It seems like one protracted and fusional *fuck of the century*.

What is striking, on the other hand, is that her story is teeming with pet names and diminutives that relate more to childhood than the bedroom. She can also cuddle endlessly with her little son, but she still lets slip that he is too much into her. Sometimes, she wonders who takes care of whom.

Olga was in inpatient psychotherapy for barely two weeks. For a moment, she let a heartwarming whirlwind blow through the ward and the group of fellow patients. In her appearance and performance, she looked like a cross between a baby and an anime girl.

Naturally, she has inherited a substantial attachment disorder from her history. Beneath a false self that functions sensibly in everyday life, there are disparate—because unintegrated—urges and post-traumatic contents like a churning undercurrent that determines her actions.

She is, as it were, defenceless in the face of it and lives in a quasi-permanent dissociated state where, in a vertical split of her personality, the 'normal' and the 'fucked-up' part remain separate.

She stayed away after the first outing weekend, and, since then, I have received several phone calls at intervals of several months to make an urgent appointment. Although, each time, she stresses how motivated she is to follow her treatment thoroughly this time, she always cancels her appointment through the hospital reception at the eleventh hour. With this kind of problem, establishing a connection that does not keep getting broken is quite a challenge. The future will show whether we will succeed in this.

## Pedro—What Women Want

This 40-something with the sex appeal of a rock star was referred by a PWGH service because he did not like having to go back home and be there alone. 'I'm going to die!' He begins to talk about how he met a girl six years before. It will be revealed later that he is said to have rescued her from prostitution. She was supposedly infertile but, a month into the relationship, she was already pregnant. She went abroad with another man in the sixth month of her pregnancy.

After a short time, this new partner dropped her back at Pedro's door. He feels outrage towards her: she thinks she can get away with everything and behaves irresponsibly. She blames her problems on others, is always on the run, and is 'constantly looking for excuses'. Meanwhile, she has already left, but their little daughter is with Pedro, although he strongly doubts that he is indeed the biological father.

For several years, he has had pain around his heart. He fears a 'heart attack' and has been examined several times for this, but there are no objectifiable abnormalities. Previously, Pedro had a relationship with an ex-prostitute whom he also allegedly liberated from the clutches of her pimps. She went to the gym and the sauna while he did the housework, and, when she abandoned him for another man, he felt abused 'even then'.

An older daughter from this relationship stays with him. His comment: 'I never change partners. I do everything for them. I get too attached'. He describes himself as kind-hearted and generous but, in the same breath, he also calls himself genial, versatile, and a workaholic. 'I work 14–16 hours daily and do the work of four people!'

Pedro is the elder of two and has a sister. His parents have worked hard all their lives. The mother is a somewhat fierce and hot-tempered woman but a 'pleasant conversationalist'. He did not see his father much; he was always working. The father is a bit on the cheeky side, but he means well. As a child, Pedro thought his father was an all-round terrific guy. 'I walked in his steps; I followed in his footsteps.' This went so far that his father said, 'You shouldn't imitate me like that'.

In his adolescence, Pedro learned that his father was not his biological father. This came as a shock, but he is immensely grateful to him for his excellent care. For the first few years of his life, his family worked in France. He was the fruit of his mother's brief affair with a Frenchman. When the family came to live in Belgium, Pedro was French-speaking. He was often bullied for this. He is even said to have been smacked for this on several occasions.

He was considered an exceptionally exemplary, sweet, excellent, and well-behaved boy. At the age of eight, he was sexually initiated by an aunt. Step by step, she led him to discover the secrets of female sexuality. It left him with a lifelong fascination with the female sex and female pleasure. He loves women 'terribly'. 'I know what women want.' 'They can't stay off my body.' Although this was clear sexual abuse, he is fierce and ardent in professing his love for this sugar aunty.

During his adolescence, he developed a strong *flower power* spirit. 'Imagine' by John Lennon was his favourite song. At 16, he had another sexual relationship, with a 30-year-old woman. She, too, taught him every possible sexual finesse, and he has since been able to get absorbed and high on making women reach orgasm. It is difficult for him to accept help, but he regularly goes on rescue missions for children and women in need.

Pedro had been in inpatient psychotherapy for over a year and, since then, has been coming on a fortnightly outpatient basis for about 15 years. At the beginning of treatment, he was not at all into psychology. His first ward meeting was memorable and illustrative—he was the only person sitting on the floor. He started singing a carnivalesque song by a local comedian in which bananas played a leading role. He had constant physical complaints and was afraid of dying of a (literally) broken heart. In various smaller and larger groups, he spoke up and commented on fellow patients and team members but was not inclined to look critically at himself.

He was a real ladies' man. Throughout his admission, he was surrounded by infatuated women who took off their clothes for him in no time, as is reportedly often the case with groupies where their idols are concerned. His numerous amorous affairs involving him and his fellow patients were well hidden because they only really came to light after he had disappeared from the clinical psychotherapy scene.

Throughout his admission, Pedro mainly acquired a cognitive view or overview of his history and the patterns that repeated themselves in it. First, he increasingly realised that he had not felt loved and accepted by either of his parents. Consequently, he always reached out for love and appreciation. He had initially looked up to his father, but there were few expressions of affection from him either. However, he was often called on by this figure for all sorts of dirty jobs or chores.

When Pedro learned he was the son of another man, his world collapsed. Why had his mother lied to him? Was he an unwanted child? Did he remind her of an episode in her life she preferred to forget? He tried to track down his father and succeeded after many attempts. He turned out to be a cross between a good-for-nothing and a rascal, and so he abandoned his plan to get to know him better for good. He did, however, develop a distinct fondness for France, which he has since visited as regularly as possible and which, in his eyes, is characterised by an indestructibly magnificent splendour.

Coming from a land bordered by Germany, he had incredibly cosy and homely memories of the Christmas period. Every year, from the beginning of December to the end of January, his home is magically transformed into half a Christmas village. He surrounds himself with several Christmas trees, hundreds of baubles and lights, stalls, and wreaths. He is trying to get a medal for being a father. He is, de facto, a single parent to both his daughters. He tries to give them a solid upbringing based on traditional family values but finds it hard to cope when they escape his power and control in their adolescent years.

Over the years, a few more downtrodden young women have passed by. He moves heaven and earth each time to get them out of the doldrums or the gutter. Even sexually, he makes it his business to satisfy their every need and desire. On closer inspection, behind his idealisation of women hides a great hatred and contempt. While he initially waxes lyrical when describing his vaginal activities and achievements, now and then, the undisguised loathing, disgust, and contempt hidden underneath also emerge. Women increasingly appear in his stories as superficial and outwardly focused airheads—orgasm-obsessed egoists who neglect their offspring.

That his weakness for women is a direct result of what was neither more nor less than sexual abuse has now become clear to him; he feels like a (after the pop group) 'Dildo Warhead' in whom user-friendliness and anger towards the female sex are united.

Pedro, meanwhile, is close to 60. He lives in an apartment building on the outskirts of a provincial town among (he says) immigrants, marginals, and social cases. He is a volunteer magistrate and ensures law and order as a kind of sheriff. He is strict but fair to the residents, whom he treats, somewhat authoritatively, like silly children.

Although he remains a woman magnet, he bitterly keeps the women at bay. He is often half a philosopher in reporting the goings-on in and around him. Having neither read nor studied, he formulates original and pertinent thoughts on human tragicomedy.

I have often quoted his saying, 'The patient is always right until he realises he is wrong'. At least he has come to that point himself. Meanwhile, he feels old and lonely but seems to find peace in the wisdom he has acquired through much hardship.

### Cindy—Whose Scenario?

This 60-something had a managerial position in a hospital and was fired a few months before she came to consult because of her alcohol problem. After all, she had repeatedly turned up at work smelling of booze. Since then, she has been 'dry' but was advised to undergo psychotherapy. Previously, she used to sneak in periods of drinking at home, averaging up to ten 'units' a day (when a patient expresses themself in these terms, an addiction problem is immediately apparent). One of her first statements: 'My husband is talking about divorce. I want everything neat and clean, and he wants all the dirt to stay'. It immediately evoked an association with a quote that adorns some mantelpieces: '*Le mariage est un duo ou un duel*'. Marriage is either a duo or a duel.

Cindy has been married for 30 years to Georges, a slightly older man who works as a nurse. They have two grown-up children, both of whom were doing fine psychologically and socio-professionally, and with whom Cindy says they have an excellent relationship.

She describes Georges as a chatterbox and a 'nag' who repeats the same thing 20 times a day. There are daily arguments over trivialities, but she says, in the same breath, 'I'm glad he's here'. She ended up with him out of a desire to get away from home and a fear of not getting off the streets. She has an older brother and a younger one. The former has done well socially, but the latter has 'failed'. Cindy describes her mother as a domineering woman who did not get along with anyone. Cindy was always well-behaved and submissive and did everything her mother expected of her. She mainly had to study from morning to night. Mother attached excessive importance to status. 'I always had to be the best. If I had achieved seventy per cent, I would have flown into the corner. I had to become a doctor and also marry a doctor.' Her father was under the mother's thumb. He was a sweet man who occasionally gave Cindy a penny without letting her mother know.

Cindy had her first boyfriend when she was 18. He was much older and did not impress Cindy's mother because of his age and lack of education, and so she broke off the relationship. Her current partner was more to her mother's liking, mainly because of his parents' 'good origins'. Her mother survived her father for a while, but she had also died a few years earlier. 'It is unfortunate the best party died first.' At the end of the intake interview, I often ask the patient about the story's moral. Cindy's answer: 'I swallow a lot'.

It's not often that a particular problem or pattern is as clear as this. Cindy immediately recognises that she and her partner went from bad to worse. She did not do her own thing in her professional career but followed her husband's wishes. Just how much she was dancing to her husband's tune was evident after just a few sessions from the fact that she entered a sexual relationship with the neighbour, mainly at his instigation. It turned out that she had to play a role in George's scenario, and that the latter delighted in first watching their erotic activities and then punishing her for them afterwards. She felt shame at this and anger. 'How willing you can be!'

That alcohol served multiple functions was soon apparent to her. It provided her with anaesthesia and forgetfulness, and it was a way of saying 'fuck' to everyone. That got her into serious trouble, and she took it lightly because it was what she deserved. She soon concluded that there were more options than divorcing George or letting him treat her like a puppet. She tried more than ever to refuse service. After barely a dozen calls, she told me she wanted to discontinue her weekly sessions. Hopefully, she realised in time that, although this meant she was divorcing someone, she was divorcing the wrong person. In exit interviews, the psychiatric hospital where I once worked asked so-called drop-out patients to reflect on their process and evolution. To everyone's surprise, their retrospective assessments proved to be broadly as favourable as those of patients who had ended their (semi)residential treatment on psychiatric and psychotherapeutic advice. Naturally, I hope the same for Cindy.

## Sofie—Converting a Mania

This young woman was referred for outpatient treatment by a neurologist with the presenting complaint of trichotillomania, which had allegedly been dragging on for about six years. 'I'm pulling hair out' (in Dutch, 'hair' is 'haar' and it means 'her' and 'hair'). Things started in her senior year of high school. She was then in a relationship that did not go well, with an Italian two years her senior. He was demanding and temperamental, and she had to do everything for him, physically and mentally.

In the face of his dominance, she behaved slavishly and docilely for several years until she cheated on him with someone else. 'I thought, Fuck you!' He then beat and locked her up. She managed to tell her parents about it and ran away from him overnight. He reportedly pursued her for over six months because this rejection hurt him.

Her trichotillomania is said to have started because of the stress caused by all this. But, apart from that, much is traditionally expected of her. For instance, she sets the bar high in her studies and wants to be the best in everything. She is now doing a second master's degree, and she wants a good job and an excellent career, with the motto 'to stand still is to regress'. She is never at rest, rushing from one thing to another. At the same time, she quickly and often feels lonely, and she is not very good at being alone. 'I have no one.'

She initially describes her parents as lovely people who play golf but are not a good match. They do a lot for her. With her mother, however, she has a 'love/hate relationship'. 'She puts a very high pressure on me. I was my mother's calling card.' Sofie looks up to her. She is hugely ambitious. According to her mother, a woman should be independent, preferably reaching the top of a company.

Her mother is said to be having an extramarital affair, and Sofie knows about it but cannot tell anyone. She considers her mother to be a calm, rational businesswoman who constantly installs herself in the role of victim and blames all difficulties on others. Her father, on the other hand, she describes as a doubter. She can speak to him more easily, however. He loves culture, art, and history. However, he has an alcohol problem and he does not have much of a say at home. An older brother is a problem child whose girl-friend unexpectedly got pregnant when he was only 18. The mother was fur-ious, while the father was more understanding. The whole family was on edge. Meanwhile, he has apparently 'found his feet' well in all areas.

Since childhood, Sofie has had migraine-like tension headaches. In primary school, she once cheated and was made an example of at school. She vividly remembers the embarrassment and humiliation. She was a very nervous child and wet the bed for a long time. 'My parents took good care of me, especially materially.' Her mother was not around much. It was mainly her father who took care of her. Her mother, she felt, was strict. Sofie had to eat everything, including what she didn't like. In addition, her mother is a slim, handsome, self-conscious woman who regularly comments on her daughter's looks and 'line'. Sofie suffers from a lot of insecurity and feelings of inferiority.

She was in weekly outpatient psychotherapy with me for about two years. I immediately 'read' her trichotillomania as a conversion phenomenon: the body expresses something from the unconscious through a linguistic symptom that needs to be deciphered. In an initial conversation, the patient usually (not yet too hampered by transference and resistance) speaks freely, often without knowing or realising what they are saying or how much truth is hidden in each word.

According to the statement above, 'I'm pulling hair/her out', I deduced from the whole context that, although she was unaware of any wrongdoing, she had been walking around with a lot of repressed and bottled-up anger for a long time. Her partner seemed to me to be a variant of the narcissistic mother who treated and controlled her as a kind of self-object.

Especially when she also began to experience, within the therapeutic relation-ship, that she was trying to 'do her best' to meet my expectations, it began to dawn on her. Over time, this chore weighed so much on her that she wanted to 'pull the plug on therapy'. When I related this to pulling *the hair* out, so to speak, the lightbulb lit up for Sofie. It would be evidence of her problem for the rest of the conversations. In each case, it provided adequate explanations for what was repeated in variations on the theme in her socio-professional life.

While the father had initially remained out of touch, she began to see him in a different light over time. His fine words and cultural and book wisdom notwithstanding, he had too little to say at home and in parenting and, as a result, had not been able to constrain the mother's imperatives sufficiently. Sofie felt emotionally let down by him (too) and started viewing him in a less idealised way. When she met an 'ordinary, good guy' and went to live with him in another province, despite her mother's opposition, she completed therapy with me.

Psychoanalytic psychotherapy is a trial-and-error undertaking. As a therapist, you form a hypothesis that is tested by (trial) interpretations. The latter can be strengthened and refined if these produce additional 'material' under associations that confirm the hypothesis. Ultimately, the patient becomes an expert in themself. They distil from symptoms and other surface phenomena the laws that determine their psychological life and, with more knowledge of internal affairs, try to draw the appropriate conclusions from this.

## Victoria—Snow White's Nightmare

Victoria was still a young woman in her mid-20s when she was referred to a PWGH service after several admissions and several years of mostly medicated outpatient treatment. She is the youngest of three daughters. Her father held a managerial position. He was a popular figure in the outside world but erratic at home. Sometimes, he was sweet and affectionate; other times, he was critical and demanding. He humiliated and belittled Victoria and was never satisfied with her excellent performance in school. From early adolescence, he commented on her appearance and occasionally invaded her bathroom and bedroom. She felt unprotected under his eyes—a piece of meat subjected to inspection every time. Yet she still had better contact with him than with her mother. She felt he was in conflict with himself and, at times, she felt some warmth and (though wordless) emotional understanding from his side.

Victoria has never had a good relationship with her mother. She is described as a vain, self-centred woman who is jealous of her daughters. Overall, Victoria has positive memories of the early years of her life. She spent much time with her loving and friendly grandparents and rode her little bike in the street. She was felt more at home with friends' parents.

She was unprepared for their move, when she was eight, to a distant region where a different language was spoken. Since then, she has never really been able to settle down. At home, she felt confined and controlled. Her sisters revolted openly by slamming doors and raising their voices, which sometimes led to their being locked in the cellar. As a result, Victoria was always relatively well-behaved and docile. However, she felt figuratively trapped in a basement. She constantly slaved away to be liked. For instance, she achieved fine results at school but had to endure an ordeal at home with every exam because of her hot-tempered father who supposedly 'helped' her with her studies but mostly made her very scared and insecure.

Physically, she was precocious and struggled a lot with this. She wanted to remain small and asexual. That felt safer. She hardly ever had boyfriends. She felt far too bad about herself for this. During her high school years, her father was diagnosed with cancer. She cared for him physically and witnessed his deterioration up close and in the most painful and intimate details. Her mother remarried afterwards, and she had a decent bond and contact with her stepfather. She studied at university and worked in the care sector for several years. She lived with a slightly older boyfriend, but she did not feel understood by him.

In a well-known simile, Freud compares the psychoanalytic process to peeling an onion. It is dismantled, from superficial to deeper layers. This is by no means a pleasant job and almost always involves the secretion of the necessary bodily fluids. A patient who found me via internet searches also said, in the first interview, that psychotherapy has to have three components—insight, behaviour, and regression. I remember being amazed that this last truth could even be discovered digitally!

All in all, I have been working with Victoria for about 15 years. She had several long-term episodes of inpatient psychotherapy in full (24-hour) admission and in day treatment. In between, there was also continuous outpatient psychotherapy, according to her evolving needs, once or twice a week. Episodically, admission within the clinical psychotherapeutic mother environment was necessary because she was prey to catastrophic fears and unbearable feelings of loneliness and abandonment. Although she never made an actual suicide attempt, she soon ended up at the emergency exit at these times.

This alternated with periods when she fought her way out and managed to bring various business initiatives to fruition. There were also prolonged periods of work resumption. She chooses her employment each time because of its warm and 'family' atmosphere, but is also disappointed in this respect. Each time, she appears to function excellently and to everyone's satisfaction. She is eager to work and takes initiative and responsibility. Gradually, however, she starts to feel abused and exploited in a professional setting where only money matters and patient care is not taken very seriously.

Initially, her story revolved mainly around the father. Although no actual incidents had occurred, his attitude towards her was emotionally and sexually transgressive, and she has often felt harassed, threatened, hurt, and humiliated by him. For example, she has unpleasant and painful memories of how he 'helped' her with maths exercises. He demanded that she understand everything immediately. This attitude made her tense and fearful of failure because he could either lash out at her furiously or mockingly and scornfully if she did not succeed immediately. Such exercises were, therefore, neither more nor less than torture for her.

She also suffered from him as a woman (in the making). She felt chased by him to the bathroom, and he commented on her physical changes during her (pre)puberty. Although she has elegant and fashionable looks, she has very low self-esteem as a woman because of this, among other things. She often feels peeped at, watched, inspected—an object or object of suffering under the male gaze.

Even in therapy, she sometimes appears to feel uncomfortable and unsafe because she is being watched. It is difficult to determine whether what she is telling me is correct. Shouldn't it be performed to my liking? However, her low self-esteem is not only related to her father. Gradually, the focus of her story shifts to the mother, who, over time, becomes the most important (because most pernicious) figure in her life.

Victoria's mother emerges from her story as a very business-focused and commercially minded woman who integrates into and moves smoothly in fashionable circles. She is beautiful and stylishly sexy and she knows just how to use her feminine assets and charms to get her way with everyone. At this stage of her therapy, the comparison with Snow White's haughty mother, who is so jealous that she wants to have her killed, is repeatedly made!

Victoria gives many examples of how her mother interferes with her hair-style, the length of her hair, her clothing (including swimming costumes), and so on. If her changing body shape is overly appreciated and highlighted by her father, then, because of her mother, the opposite is systematically the case.

Then comes the most extended, most challenging, and most profound phase of her trial, during which massive feelings of abandonment, rage, and depression engulf her. Countless memories of her mother's unloving treatment emerge. How she lay motionless and alone in her cot and had to bottle-feed herself. How few clothes and even fewer toys she got from her mother. When they went shopping together, the mother bought a lot for herself but nothing for her daughter. When she (allegedly) bought accessories or jewellery for Victoria, they inevitably ended up in her mother's wardrobe, and so on. Examples of both material and affective neglect are legion. During this period, she is completely helpless and vitally dependent on a maternal environment for months. Intensive nursing and nurturing are necessary to help her get through this deep valley in one piece. Her (child's) room is teeming with ghosts during this period. The mother is an evil witch who haunts her. When she leaves the safety of the clinical psychotherapeutic environment at weekends or for out-of-home activities, she is terrified of running into her mother as if she were a witch in front of whom she feels totally naked, defenceless, and at her mercy.

After this deep regression period, she came back in fits and starts. She came to weekly outpatient treatment for about two years. She built a stable partner relationship with a kind and understanding new partner she met at the beginning of her treatment, and that has endured through much adversity.

Numerous anecdotes show that Victoria is very good with children, but she nevertheless doubted for a long time whether she was a 'good mother'. Even before puberty, she had gynaecological complaints. One of her ovaries was removed when she was still a child, and she expressed several fears about not being able to have children later on. Neither parent paid much attention to this. From puberty onwards, she had challenging periods, which meant she barely made it to school. Hardly any care was given to this either. When she failed to get pregnant naturally, and given her 'biological clock' and her ever-increasing desire for children, the couple started fertility treatment at two university centres. With all the nasty side effects of hormone treatment and commuting to university cities at all possible and impossible times, it has been a veritable road to Calvary for her and her partner, which, moreover, yielded nothing. She felt heartless and treated mechanically, like an incubator, by doctors who, in her eyes, all displayed rather prominent narcissistic traits.

At long last, she was diagnosed (very belatedly!) with endometriosis and had to undergo a radical hysterectomy. In many ways, this meant a death blow for her. We needed about two years of two sessions a week to overcome this blow.

In old terms, such surgery (where both uterus and ovaries are removed) is called a 'castration'. Of course, it is not only men who have castration anxiety and/or can be castrated and/or feel castrated, primarily when the penis acquires a more symbolic meaning via the Lacanian phallus as that which we can never be or have (enough) to (fully) satisfy the desire of the great Other. I refer to my previous book for this, as I will limit myself to Victoria's clinic here.

First, Victoria was angry and sad because of the negligence she accused her parents and doctors of. How could everyone be so smug, and how could everyone have overlooked her pain? Second, for once and for all, this meant the death sentence for her desire to have children. The possibility of starting a family of her own and thus making some reparation for her own missed family happiness was—she felt cruelly—taken away from her. She undertook various initiatives to realise 'the next best thing' (adoption, fostering, and so on). Still, she came up against lengthy procedures and many requirements, including a 'blank' psychiatric history, so that her courage for such an undertaking plummeted. Any dealings with mothers and/or children were always extremely difficult for her. Indeed, the transient joy she could derive from interacting with children never outweighed the associated suffering and loss. Because her work brought her into frequent contact with young mothers and children, it was with great pain that she had to give up the substantively stimulating managerial position she had achieved there. On all levels, this left her feeling empty-handed.

Last but not least, through and underneath all this was the subtext of a mother who had robbed and deprived her of her most precious potential. Indeed, for Victoria, the verdict of permanent childlessness implied both an unbearable loss and lack and an indigestible 'defeat' by her mother. How much had she 'fought' to get 'there'? For a long time, she was bitter about what years of psychotherapy had brought her. All her efforts were (literally) fruitless. Exemplary achievements notwithstanding, she was not rewarded.

For instance, some patients have something like the 'basic fault' Michael Balint discussed. They have missed as a basis the simultaneously ordinary and extraordinary (because hardly to be found elsewhere) godsend of motherly love. This problem can be as intractable as rising damp from the cellar. It is an early childhood trauma, and it can long feel like an abyssal crater that makes it hard ever to be grounded enough. She was regularly close to acts of despair and, over the years, she had to be pulled to safety several times to avoid fatal 'accidents'. Variations on the theme of abandonment, rage, and depression in connection with various 'narcissistic' figures (including me) kept coming up at length. Meanwhile, Victoria recognises that she will have to make do with sublimation. After some experiments in more commercial roles, she gradually regained joy in the labour of caring for her patients who are, after all, (like herself) children in distress. At her request, psychotherapy has since been reduced to a fortnightly frequency.

## Wilma—Psychology of Prey

This 50-year-old woman immediately pounced in the introductory interview:

> I live alone. I have good children, sons-in-law and grandchildren. I have good friends. But something has happened that has completely upset me. I am in shock. I can't live with it. I went to a physiotherapist because of chronic back pain. The first visit was not too bad. At the second consultation, however, something happened. Instead of cracking me, he moved on to sexual acts. I am only half aware of what happened. He has gone too far. I feel abused and assaulted. Why did I let him do me? I can't tell anyone. I live with a lie, with a secret. I live a double life. I am having such a hard time!

On the one hand, she calls this therapist a charlatan. She ranks him as a *mala fide* person who did not behave deontologically or professionally. On the other hand, she feels very embarrassed and guilty. She would like to categorically forget this experience. 'I would like to erase them from my hard drive.'

Wilma was married for about ten years to a man quite a bit older than her. She has two daughters from this marriage. After that, she had three other long-term relationships. The first was with the brother of her first husband, with whom she was in love for the first time. However, he put increasing pressure on her, making her feel chained and wanting to tear herself away.

In the second long-term relationship, she experienced the greatest love. However, he fell seriously ill shortly after they met, and she took care of him for five years. He was a true 'soulmate'. After his death, she experienced her first major depression. 'I missed Hugo. *I needed* a father figure.' Her last relationship lasted the longest. In her own words, she threw herself into this relationship to avoid grieving for Hugo. She has been single again for more than five years.

Wilma is the second of four children. Her mother is a housewife. 'Now I find her loving, but I found her hard as a child. I received little affection from her. She ruled with a hard hand and never showed understanding when I needed it.' Her father was a plumber. He was away from home a lot. She hardly knew him. He was kind of under her mother's thumb. As a child, Wilma loved to play a lot. She sang, recited poetry, and was top of her class at school. However, she often felt excluded because she was 'too pretty'. She loved going to girl scouts. Then, she was away from home. Her mother did not allow her to pursue higher studies. She was always frustrated about this.

Sexual trauma can occur within or outside a relationship of trust. More-over, it can have incestuous implications when it involves an asymmetrical and dependent relationship (e.g. teacher–pupil, therapist–patient). In addition it is always grafted on a history that determines its impact and meaning.

That the physiotherapist abused her is also a fact for the patient. However, this does not prevent her from feeling very ashamed and guilty. Shame affects the self or the whole person. It has a massive impact: the person concerned would like to sink into the ground or disappear off the face of the Earth rather than feel naked and humiliated. Guilt strikes more at a specific aspect or act of the person. There is a tendency or possibility to make amends.

With regard to Wilma's feelings, there are, by all means, proximal and possibly distal reasons. Proximal reasons can be understood as follows: by definition, a person is unprepared for trauma. They feel, to a greater or lesser extent, bewildered, dumbfounded, paralysed, rooted to the ground, knocked off the hand of God. When they are (as Wilma herself calls it) 'in shock', they can no longer react adequately. They cannot fight or flee. They freeze and/or submit in an automatic (prompted by the desire to preserve life and limb) 'collaboration'.

Once they have made such a mistake, they are trapped. They have done wrong, so they must suffer the 'punishment' that comes with it. Behold the fatal (psycho)logic that kicks in with many sexual traumas. It was also evident in Wilma's case.

But those who work psychotherapeutically can also search for deep, more distal layers. Why exactly did this happen to Wilma? Indeed, the predator does not choose this or that prey by chance. It has a 'nose', as it were, for the person who lends themself best as a victim. In doing so, it unerringly reads the language of a body that betrays (often unconsciously and unknowingly) 'true' feelings or desires. Are there no underlying desires or fantasies at work that help fuel Wilma's feelings of guilt and shame? According to Freud, doesn't the gospel tell us to look for the famous Oedipus complex? If this were the case with Wilma at all, such exploration would be appropriate and fruitful if and only if the trauma, as such, has been sufficiently processed. Otherwise, an exploratory approach (if not *Hineininterpretierung*) risks fur-ther fuelling already present and unbearable feelings of guilt. It is possibly because her underlying father hunger was addressed inappropriately or pre-maturely that Wilma attempted suicide after several weeks of admission. Her attempt was fortunately foiled. The psychotherapist would still be able to make up for his lack of understanding and rapport with Wilma.

Only in psychotherapeutic work afterwards did she feel sufficiently believed and recognised in her position as victim. It took more than a year of further outpatient psychotherapy before she could focus on the fledgling interaction with her physiotherapist. This time, without self-blame or condemnation, she could recognise in it, through a few close-ups, the *Gestalt* of both the phsyiotherapist and her much-missed father. Was it this fatal combination that had left her so defenceless to his unexpected manoeuvre? Quite possibly, but that does not make an abuse victim a guilty party!

## Conny—a Psychological Cancer

This 45-year-old woman was referred after multiple admissions to PWGH services and psychiatric hospitals, where treatment was stopped owing to persistent suicidality and self-harm. She is an only child. Her mother is a blue-collar worker. She is described as highly authoritative, hot-tempered, and aggressive/violent. For example, Conny was dragged by her hair through the kitchen and locked in the coal shed by her mother. As a child, Conny always felt unwanted; she felt abused as a kind of 'white slave' and was used as a maid-of-all-work.

Her father is an office worker. He is described as a great absentee and was not a hugger. She further characterises him as strict and punctual. He was initially somewhat put on a pedestal by Conny, 'idolised'. After puberty, she discovered that her father was a transvestite. More than once, she caught him in his mother's clothes. He became a sexually insecure figure for her. The abuse by her mother only effectively started from the age of eight. Fortunately, throughout, she could cling to a German shepherd dog who was her support and with whom she could share all her emotional distress. Besides all this, there was also weekly sexual abuse by her paternal grandfather between the ages of 6 and 12, resulting in various post-traumatic symptoms, broken trust, and sexual aversion.

Conny did higher studies and invested a lot in work. After her children were born, more acute conflict arose between work and family (wanting to be a good mother). For the last seven years, she has worked full-time in education. After four years of courtship, she married a darling man. The couple has two sons. The eldest is cuddly, 'he hangs on me'; the youngest is said to have ADHD and ASD.

There have been massive sexual problems since the desire for children was satisfied. Conny cannot tolerate any physical contact. For years, there has been major depression, passive-regressive behaviour, flights into bed, and very severe and persistent para-suicidal self-harming. She exhibits rational, solid control, and a wide gap exists between her outside and inside. She can appear intense, gritty, and cheerful while feeling like hell inside, haunted and tormented by a haunting inner object that can be understood as a conglomeration of mother and grandfather. She calls it the 'brain picker' and she repeatedly draws pictures as if it were some hermaphrodite monster eating her from within.

Conny went through several years of clinical psychotherapeutic treatment. Episodically, she had to be continuously monitored for months and depended on intensive care. With some physiological issues, the patient is put into an artificial coma, and vital functions are supported or taken over by life support systems.

Psychotherapy, especially with this type of difficulty, is a harrowing undertaking that only proceeds optimally with full consciousness and certainly without general anaesthesia. In some psychotherapeutic operations, the entire life force must come from the therapists or outside the patient; after all, internal destructive forces (which may or may not also be understood as a death drive) rule.

Conny made numerous suicide attempts during her treatment and had to be transferred to a nearby emergency department every so often because of severe self-injury, frequently accompanied by near-fatal blood loss. Thus, for a long time, she tried to evacuate her unbearable psychological suffering in a 'mute' manner, without recourse to (help from) others.

Besides tolerance and empathy, compassion on the therapist's part is required. They may be inclined to evacuate (the suffering of) the patient (as was the case in previous counselling) but must be prepared to suffer with the patient to help carry and digest raw drive and trauma. The extraordinary emotional care that can only be provided by a clinical psychotherapeutic mother environment's entire team is vital. The purpose was to restore and build basic safety and trust and to continuously process the inner struggle between good and bad inner (partial) objects. This is in addition to the long and arduous process of digesting traumatic re-experiences.

The treatment was seriously hampered and complicated by the fact that Conny was left by her husband (who had been very understanding for a long time). Although many conflicts arose around the division of already limited financial and material resources, the divorce proceeded constructively. The fact that the partner always correctly allowed standard visitation arrangements to continue as much as possible commanded respect and admiration.

Despite the worries and heartbreak, Conny, too, could explicitly appreciate this. She tried to be a 'good mother' as much as possible. Nevertheless, her difficulties weighed heavily on the children. 'Mum can only express her love with trips and presents', they were told in conversation. The children suffered from the mother's severe psychopathology rather than the divorce. Both received counselling from our hospital's service for children of psychiatric patients. Both were in psychotherapy themselves for quite a long time.

Throughout her treatment, Conny maintained contact with her former outpatient psychotherapist. Since she left the hospital about three years ago, she has had sessions there twice a week and comes to me fortnightly for psychiatric and process counselling. She has since bought a home, does voluntary work, and receives home-based counselling thanks to the mobile psychiatric team.

Partly as a result of the long-term use of atypical neuroleptics, she gained dozens of kilograms. She was now undergoing bariatric surgery, resulting in the normalisation of her weight. At their request, I recently saw the now adolescent children. They have a lot of reflective and mentalising abilities, but the elder child, in particular, is still suffering from manifest parentification. The younger one is considering breaking contact with his mother sooner or later. He fears that, at some point, it might become too much for him.

For a lot of psychological problems, a comparison with cancer treatment holds. The patient is prey to malignant processes that can metastasise to the furthest reaches of the psyche. The oncologist pulls out all the stops to reduce or contain proliferation. Even in the best case, the patient never returns to a state where (fear of) cancer is absent. Even with the best and most sophisticated approach, oncology care must sometimes lose out. In the end, sooner or later, all patients die. Meanwhile, ethical care and diligence are required. Thankfully, the days are gone when a terminal cancer patient ended up alone in a multi-person room and—as if they were a leper—everyone stayed away and/or tried to avoid any conversation about prognosis. With equally malignant psychological processes, a humane and high-quality approach often slips far behind.

## Vadim—a Bald Samson

This 30-something was referred for therapy after withdrawal from alcohol and sedatives. He has been hospitalised a dozen times for this purpose, including under the statute of forced treatment. By his admission, he suffers from alcohol dependence, mood swings, anxiety, and depression. He staggers from one hospital to another.

Vadim is employed in education but has no steady job. He has been in a relationship with a divorced mother of three for about seven years, but, because of his toxicomania, they are in a living-apart-together relationship. He has good contact with the children, but, partly because he has been in all kinds of states, his girlfriend has become distrustful to the point of controlling. Vadim finds it hard to be alone and feels anxious and trapped in his own home. He is unsatisfied with himself and feels he has already squandered many opportunities.

Vadim is the youngest of three children. He calls his relationship with his parents very poor. They had a flourishing butcher's shop and retired to the coast in their 50s. His father passed away shortly after this. He is said to have been an anxious, even people-shy, introverted man. On the other hand, he was also proud and jealous. He spoiled Vadim materially but was never concerned with his youngest son. 'I never received love from him.'

His mother was already well into her 40s when Vadim was born (unwanted). She always followed his father in everything but was emotionally and sexually very frustrated and turned to Vadim with her unmet needs. He was her support, crutch, and confidant. Until adolescence, he regularly shared a bed with his mother. She sexually abused him several times, seeking with him the satisfaction (up to coitus) she did not find with her father. He describes himself as the 'lubricant' at home. 'I had to keep quiet, get good marks and fill mother's hole.'

He was a good student but an absolute loner. He felt he did not belong anywhere. Consequently, he carried an incestuous secret like a leaden burden, which he could not or did not dare to share with anyone. From puberty onwards, he became more popular. He put on a swagger, grew his hair, and acted like a muscular big boy. Inwardly, he remained insecure and fearful of failure, with strongly fluctuating moods. During his higher education, he started drinking excessively and abusing tranquillisers and sleeping pills.

Vadim has been married for a dozen years and has a daughter from this marriage whom he no longer sees as a result of a hostile divorce that left him bankrupt. In his opinion, his ex was not what she first seemed. He sought warmth and affection from her, but she was an ambitious career woman for whom only financial gain mattered. 'As soon as I started to struggle emotionally, she dropped me like a brick.'

The gap between reason and feeling can sometimes be awe-inspiring. Vadim had two sides. He was emotionally on point at times, with a clear view of his twisted parents and history. Then again, he was a vessel of raw, unintegrated, and unmentalised (sexual and aggressive) temper. He sometimes tried to smooth it with vast amounts of alcohol. In trauma, it does often happen that failing repression (the not-forgetting) is 'resolved' by massive substance use. Virtually all brain activity can, after all, only be flattened chemically.

For Vadim, however, this just added fuel to the fire, and he ended up in fights or frantically turning his home into a mess or battlefield. He did know what was proper and healthy and could say it all well and explain it convincingly. However, when it came down to it, he could not live up to these acceptable words and values and, in his own words, felt completely 'fucked up'.

Throughout the conversations, he became well aware of the scope and impact of the incestuous relationship with his mother. She had taken him to a no-man's land beyond all limits and enslaved him to a toxic pleasure. It managed to put him into a kind of intoxication that made him feel great and all-powerful, elevated above everyone (including his father).

The other side of this coin involved great feelings of shame and guilt, as well as abandonment, anger, and depression. Was Mother concerned with him, or was he just a 'Samson' (the name of a dildo he once cynically appointed himself with) to her? Father, on the other hand, had relinquished responsibility, as he had been unable to restrain either the mother or himself. In this context, he quoted a verse by Herman de Coninck: 'Give me limits, make me small'.

Vadim was in inpatient psychotherapy for just under a year. There, he gained an overview and understanding of his problems. Still, there were also a few alcoholic excursions during admission that culminated in sex and violence and even led to police intervention. With his acting-out behaviour, he was, in a sense, asking to come into contact with the arm of the law. He denounced his 'one night stands in the cell' in that context.

Somewhat prematurely, he completed his treatment at the start of a new school year. Despite an erratic CV full of gaps, he had sold himself well again. However, he failed to show up after a few scheduled consultations. I learned through word of mouth, about a year later, that he was forcibly hospitalised following yet another alcoholic coma.

## Mattias—Torrero Therapy

Mattias is a 30-something with the looks of a matador. He applies for admission, saying he wants to dig. 'I want a different mindset. I am prone to addiction. I want different twists in my head.' He describes himself as very creative and emotional, a dreamer with difficulty dealing with authority: 'I always think I am the best, that I am always right'. He spontaneously says he struggles to get along with 'short-sighted people'. Although it will later be revealed that he is not qualified for this, he describes himself as an interior decorator. He has never worked long for the same employer. 'I always quit on my own.' Either it didn't click with the boss, or he was too perfectionist and couldn't add enough water to the wine.

The reason for his admission is that, for the umpteenth time, he had an accident while drunk. The car was a write-off, and a passenger friend was quite seriously injured. 'I have been in a lot of wrecks.' Mattias is back living with his mother and her boyfriend. He lived independently but found it hard to get his bearings. He has had a few relationships. In one, he and his partner loved each other to death. Yet he cheated on her several times, and she herself ran off with someone else after a few years. In others, he lacked security in the relationship, or the relationship broke down owing to his drinking.

Mattias is the eldest of three. A younger brother and sister have no manifest problems and have 'made their way' in life to a greater or lesser extent. His parents divorced when he was on the threshold of adolescence. He has had no contact with his father since then. This is a significant loss because 'we had a wonderful father who did everything for us'. However, since he has a new partner, the father no longer looks after his children. Mattias once went to his door. He saw his father's shadow behind the glass, but the door was not opened. 'I am like air to him.' It is painful and entirely incomprehensible for Mattias. There is manifest sorrow and anger around this.

His mother works hard and long hours in the hospitality industry. Mattias describes her as a very driven woman who makes her many dreams come true and whom he can count on. In the same breath, he says she often changes her mind at the last minute. She constantly wants to plan and arrange her life, and so he perceives her as too oppressive and frequently lies to her about everything.

From childhood, he lived immersed in a fantasy world of his own. He could spend hours with all kinds of creative things in his room. On the other hand, he struggled in the group and was only 'on the same level' with a few. He felt different and superior, was very curious, and had broad interests. He never coped with 'superficiality and stupidity'.

From adolescence, he smoked cannabis almost daily and also used speed and cocaine daily for many years. There was also copious and disinhibited drinking of alcohol. He lives more or less continuously above his means, piles up unpaid bills, and is still regularly given extra money by his mother, who also pays his traffic fines. He drives hundreds of kilometres to get fresh air at the beach and can only cook with the most exotic and/or exclusive ingredients that must be bought in various specialist shops.

In a way, Mattias does realise something is wrong with his character. He even has an idea of *what* is wrong with it. He knows he has trouble with boundaries, limitations, and authority. He drinks too much and also seeks intense intoxication in broader terms; he needs love and attention and gets easily frustrated when not everything goes to his liking. He has been in clinical psychotherapy with us for about six months, and it soon becomes clear to him what has grown askew, where, and why in his development. The absent father, the boundless mother, the splendid isolation of Fantasyland that he has wallowed in since childhood.

Classically, the patient first has complaints and symptoms they want to eliminate as quickly and smoothly as possible. Preferably, the cure is based on a prescription that they merely have to follow or swallow. We then try to infect them with the virus of curiosity. What do my problems mean? What is behind or beneath them? When did the first signs of problems occur? What feelings or sensitivities are repeating themselves? What are the roots of these phenomena? The longest and most challenging part of the psychotherapeutic process is working through. You already know what is going on and why, but it nevertheless persists in an almost demonic way.

Mattias became the wonder boy of the group. He won the hearts of many female patients with his tricks, flaunted his emotional sensitivity, and appealed to many of them with his mischievous charm. In no time, a romantic relationship with a fellow group member developed. Despite our numerous confrontations and interpretations, there was no stopping them, and they rapidly became an official couple, even in their respective home environments, rendering further clinical psychotherapeutic treatment ineffective and preparing both for outpatient psychotherapy.

After their discharge from the hospital, it soon became apparent that the fellow patient unknowingly took the torch from Mattias's mother. She was 'crazy' about Mattias, was enchanted by his physical beauty but also by his sexual and other achievements, and she provided abundant material and financial support for a long time. We are now some five years later. In the meantime, Mattias changed employers several more times, and there were several traffic violations and accidents while drunk. This time, the new partner helped pay for the costs.

Mattias visits me and a psychologist very irregularly. Whenever he makes a mistake, he buys time and goodwill by supposedly repenting and being motivated to 'work on himself'.

His partner, on the other hand, is continuously in well-run psychotherapy. She started and completed studies in counselling and is now working for in-home care. After much mess and misery, she put an end to her relationship with Mattias. What she feared (also out of jealousy) has now happened: he has already found a new partner. Her scathing and bitter words: 'History repeats itself: a bullfighter and a stupid goat!'

## François—between Orgy and Meeting

This 30-something was referred from a PWGH, where he had been hospitalised with alcohol intoxication over a month before.

> I was beside myself. I blew everything up. I still have my job and my girl-friend. I don't care about anything anymore. Nothing means anything to me anymore. I am tired from living, and I haven't lived yet. I have had everything. I am never happy, never satisfied. There is no constancy in my life. All that I try doesn't succeed. I've had a few relationships—and a few jobs. I am also an alcoholic but have been sober for three years. I had relapsed and was hospitalised as a result. I got married at the age of nine-teen, two months after my mother's suicide. I found her. She had hanged herself. My girlfriend was living with us at the time. Her parents would not accept me. My world collapsed. From the age of thirteen, I already started drinking a lot, and this increased sharply after my marriage. I also used marijuana, cocaine and XTC, but especially a lot of poppers almost daily. After a few weeks, I started going to bars. I had a lot of one-night stands. Also, with men or with transsexuals. A man and a woman in one person: that interested me. At twenty, I had already made my first suicide attempt with alcohol and medication. I had caught my wife with another man in my bed. Afterwards, we started partner swapping. Our relationship bled to death. Around age 25, I got divorced for real. Then, I met another woman who was eight years older. We stayed together for several years. I always kept on swerving. I wanted to push them into swinging. I had several short relationships with prostitutes. I am also currently in a relationship with a prostitute. I have been with a 15-year-older woman for five years. Making love is no longer possible. I can't give love. I wouldn't say I like myself; I am at odds with myself. I don't know what I want. Everything with me is based on pleasure and sex. I have to slow down. I still go to bars, clubs and saunas. They want to bond with me, but I don't want a bond. I can't be alone, and I can't be together.

François is the youngest of three sons. His mother was a housewife. He describes her as very well-behaved and caring. She would never hurt anyone. She was, however, a bit naive or even simple. 'We had a very close relation-ship.' Until adolescence, they would lie on the sofa watching television in each other's arms. 'I found that blissful.' His father was a blue-collar worker and is described as very closed and bitter. Contact is very strained. 'We don't talk to each other.'

As a child, he was very closed off, was quite heavy, and was bullied for this.

> I didn't feel accepted anywhere. Mother was over-protective, and I was bored. I was not allowed to join the youth movement at camp. I couldn't occupy myself with anything and had few toys. We had a mother but no father. He was always away and working. He only came home to complain.

Mother had to be 'father and mother at the same time'. From puberty onwards, François became very angry and rebellious towards those in power and their 'unfairness'. He could not stomach injustice. In his eyes, many a boss at work was a 'domineering bastard', who himself did not do his job correctly but constantly hoodwinked his subordinates. In addition, by his own admission, he led a dissolute life. He was afraid of liking someone. In his relationships, he wanted physical and mental submission.

François was in clinical psychotherapy with us for about a year. In the beginning, he was very messy, verging on neglectful. He was, as they say, hanging on by a thread. He seemed constantly under the influence, even though all toxicological tests were and remained negative. He also had something very feminine about him. As only one of two men in the treatment group, he wallowed in the realm of women. He bonded quickly and indulged in the emotional care of our maternal environment.

It gradually became clear to him that he had remained very much fixated on the primordial mother. His frenetic sexual activity was mainly motivated by oral and fusion strivings. It was not genitally organised but exhibited polymorphic perverse panoply. He combined devout devotion with passionate rapture towards his successive and sometimes simultaneous romantic partners. The fact that he indulged in strangulation sex could be related to the way his mother had committed suicide. We understood it as repeatedly failing attempts to reunite with his lost mother. Indeed, the close relationship with his mother had had an intoxicating and toxic effect on him. He had become addicted to these blisses, and they were at the root of his sex and substance dependence. The father had relinquished responsibility. Instead of an ally who could help him break free from his mother and become a man, he remained an apprehensive stranger against whom he rebelled. Time and again, he wanted to be ecstatically absorbed by a hermaphroditic parental figure.

Somewhat against expectations, his treatment proceeded without much hassle (at least within the hospital). For instance, he did not throw himself into a relationship with a fellow patient, nor did any major substance abuse problems arise during his admission. His fellow patients and team appreciated him for his emotional sensitivity. He raised all kinds of sexual content in the group without much hesitation, which also helped loosen others' tongues on the subject. Particularly towards me as an attending psychiatrist, there was a solid idealising transference that persisted for years after admission. From a distant province, he would regularly come to visit me and discuss stumbling blocks in his walk of life.

After treatment, François remained in the world of bars and brothels but ended up on the other side of the bar. He ran an establishment himself, had a very close and emotional relationship with the madam of the house, and took care, like a pasha, of the various prostitutes passing through. He set himself up as their protector and was able to eject sporadic troublemakers without the use of force because of his quiet firmness. It was remarkable how his 'business' was run with a sober and businesslike attitude, just as if it were a chicken farm. In neighbouring brothels and rendezvous houses, he indulged in orgies. We could understand them as an intoxicating bacchanal where the boundaries between self and love object blurred and where he surrendered anonymously and selflessly to various body parts and orifices where multiple forms of rhythmic stimulation provided him with a hot intoxication of pleasure.

He will never become the ideal son-in-law, but his psychological abilities have evolved considerably. He once gave me a photograph that I have kept to this day. He brought it to the interview like a dream that sometimes seems to have been dreamt especially for the therapist. It is a Polaroid of a pigeon sitting on a wall at dusk. It forms a line that traverses the picture plane diagonally, separating light from darkness.

The image is an apt illustration and visualisation of his psyche. He is on the edge between day and night, upper- and underworld, life and death, this side and that side of the law. He is as innocent as a dove but wants to plunge into the depths like a kamikaze pilot. It is an image full of tenderness and violence, Eros and Thanatos. We then devoted an entire session to discussing the picture. It has since adorned the mantelpiece of my office (alongside numerous other self-made gifts from patients). François looks at it (also literally) at every meeting. It is like a monument that seems to have sealed the moment of our meeting forever. It sometimes feels to him as if his bond with me is stronger than that with his dying mother.

## Jacob—the Robin Hood Complex

Jacob is around 30 when we meet and almost as skinny as a concentration camp inmate. His first words:

> I'm not doing it anymore. I have mood swings. My life is a mess. I want structure in my life. I want to break away from my mother. There is a kind of unhealthy symbiotic state between us. There is a mutual total dependence, especially on my part. I wander around. I have difficulties taking responsibility, except for others. For my responsibility, I am on the

run. I am fiercely emaciated. My eating habits are out of balance. I do things I know I can't do. There is a split between thinking and doing. I would do anything to commit suicide. I get carried away.

Jacob is the second of three children. He is back living with his mother. After studying classical humanities, he enrolled in higher education but did not complete it. During his studies, he spent much time in marginal environments, which had a strange fascination for him. He says he loves nightlife and the 'underbelly' of society. A contemporary Flemish rapper calls this the magnetism of the gutter.

On several occasions, Jacob became entangled in relationships with women in need, to whom he turned confidant. He also volunteered in Africa for several months and fell in love with another aid worker there. She struggled with depression and finally committed suicide. Since then, he has been in outpatient treatment for many years. He has also had several long-term psychiatric admissions for depression and suicidal tendencies, the latter within a (university) clinical psychotherapy setting. Following what was considered a severe premeditated suicide attempt, he was discharged from there and referred for further help in his region.

He has never really worked. He has, however, helped a lot in his father's business, where he dealt with administration. He describes his mother as contradictory: she would attract and repel him. On the one hand, she did indeed constantly draw Jacob towards herself. For instance, she spoke ill of his father, complaining about his aggressiveness and excessive sexual demands. However, when, 'point blank', she joined his father, Jacob felt cheated, rejected, and abandoned by her.

His father died a few months before. He speaks of him with admiration and awe but also with veiled criticism and anger. The father was a successful wholesaler. He did not obey rules and laws too closely. He was cheerful and friendly, a man of the world with whom Jacob was often 'on tour'. Mainly, when Jacob was still small, their father exhibited violent behaviour, drank too much, and had several car accidents. Jacob saw him as a dominant figure. His will was law. On the other hand, he was very creative and always found something new.

In one of the first conversations, he describes a scene that is brought up repeatedly over many years of treatment, the full scope and meaning of which gradually becomes clear. When Jacob was little, there were many parental quarrels and tensions. He often had trouble sleeping and felt he had to stand guard in the stairwell. He felt responsible and wanted to keep the peace. For instance, he vividly remembers a violent scene between his parents that took place on the stairs. His father shouted and ranted, but there were few blows. His mother was naked and pressed against Jacob, distraught. It was a moment he cherished. He felt simultaneously big and powerful but also fearful of reprisals from his father. Great was his surprise when, the following day, his parents sat at the breakfast table together, giggling and joking.

Some 15 years have since passed. Jacob was continuously in psychotherapy: two years of clinical psychotherapy, four years of group psychotherapy, and then several years of individual therapy. He has since undergone training, worked in the care sector for several years, married, and moved to another region. He has since been with a psychotherapist in the area and still comes to me monthly for process counselling.

We have already uncovered the same pattern in several variations on the theme. During his admission period, he remained in contact with several fellow patients. He cast himself as their support and advocate and had 'in-depth conversations' with them. In veiled terms, he criticised my therapeutic approach to his former colleagues.

At almost every consultation, he had a book he had been reading in the waiting room. These are serious psychoanalytic and literary classics he often quotes during the sessions. One of his idols is James Ellroy. He particularly likes his autobiography, *My Dark Places*. Other greats also pass by. He looks up to these father figures, tries to fathom them and belittle their work.

This showdown with the admired also plays out towards me. Gradually, he becomes aware that he is always standing up for children and women in need and trying to rescue them from the grip of (in his eyes) power-hungry people. This means he always ends up in the eye of the storm, often 'catching the gust' or losing out himself, and then finds it hard to stand (his) loss.

He regularly compares himself to Robin Hood, the scheming hero who stands up for the weak, goes to war against the sheriff, and hooks Lady/Maid Marian. You may not have to be Sigmund Freud to see a variation of the Oedipus complex in it. Incestuous desires and a specific tendency towards parricide are, as we know, its standard ingredients.

Over the years, he has varied this theme. He compares himself to Robin, Batman's right-hand man, to the squire of a knight, but also to Hamlet, who almost goes mad with doubt and indecision while, or because, he wants to kill the man who shares his mother's bed.

Only by understanding how your history grips you can you (if desired) free yourself from it. This is desirable because it often exposes a kind of existential scenario. It is a fundamental fantasy that structures your whole life and personality. Below or beyond it, there is nothing.

What will be left of Jacob if he abandons his mission? He chooses (but this time consciously) to identify with it. It's all *vanitas*, after all—vanity. The pursuit of wind. With all his literary baggage, he often refers to Shakespeare's dramas. On life, for instance, he quotes Hamlet: it is a tale told by an idiot, full of sound and fury, signifying nothing.

However, this realisation is not so terrible. In Jacob's case, for instance, it paradoxically leads to a (literally vital) melancholy. He also sometimes explicitly adopts a tragic position. In Melanie Klein's view, in a schizoid-paranoid position, we place all evil outside ourselves; in the depressive position, we situate (the source of) evil within ourselves. Only in the tragedy does evil become a category for which, in a sense, no one is really to blame. There is, then, a conflict because of the different 'parties', both understandable and legitimate positions or interests. Jacob does seem to want to be permanently delighted (Jacques Lacan: *jouissance*) in the position of a tragic hero.

## Rose—Fill It with Sand

'When I was fourteen, my father killed himself by hanging. I stayed at home for one week and then continued my studies.' Such are the first words of a 30-year-old woman referred from a PWGH. She has a very joyless appearance. When she smiles, it is not warmly. She comes across as severe and difficult. There is also something dull in the way she speaks. Something seems to have died in her.

Rose is the youngest of three children. Her older brother and sister have 'got the better of it'. As far as I can tell, they are doing fine on all counts. 'They don't talk about it at all anymore.' Her father worked in the care sector. She describes him as a very humorous, universally liked figure. His patients were full of praise for him. He had a full social life and often performed as a musician. As a father, he was 'strict but fair', especially towards going out. Rose went everywhere with him; she could cuddle with him. 'I cannot be angry with him for what he did; because of his depressed state, he was no longer my father.' She is convinced that, 'Father still sees us. I still speak to him'. There are multiple noted psychiatric antecedents of depression on his side of the family.

Her mother is an office worker. She is described as a powerful woman who has endured many difficulties. Rose can go to her for anything and feels entirely at ease with her. After her father died, she asked to sleep in the same bed as her. This lasted about a year. To this day, she is very close to her. She shares everything with her and has no secrets from her.

From childhood, Rose was clean, tidy, and responsible. She performed well at school and had many friends, boys and girls. Since the age of 18, she has been in a steady relationship with a man who is much older and with whom she feels 'safe'. Because of health problems, she had to quit the job she loved. Since then, she has been employed 'just barely' several times, which has been challenging. There were gradually increasing symptoms of anxiety and depression, with fears that she might suffer the same fate as her father. She had already made a serious suicide attempt as well.

Based on the first conversation, we can infer that Rose has not processed her father's sudden and unexpected death. It is as if it happened only yesterday. Emotionally, she seems to deny his absence. She is still stricken and in shock. Immediately after this traumatic loss, it was 'business as usual'. The crater caused by her father's suicide? Fill it with sand! Her mourning remained raw. Little psycholgical work was done around it.

The people around her do not seem to have minced too many words concerning the loss. There is denial and so-called hypomanic defence in the form of a flight forward. The grief has been split off and has not become integrated. Her environment did not sufficiently mirror Rose's feelings and, therefore, did not give Rose enough of a (mentalised) place. On the other hand, there was a regression in which the rebellion, individuation-separation, and sexuality inherent in adolescence stalled as if the paternal ban on going out had become a kind of standing order.

Rose began to lean on her mother, somewhat tearfully. What do you do when you have already lost one eye? She developed a false self that ostensibly kept up with her peers (studies, relationships, etc.), based on which she could keep up 'appearances' for many years. When she encountered a professional obstacle, she was overtaken by her shadow. The piece of her that had stopped seeing the light of day came to the fore. In addition to these psychological factors, some predispositions needed to be considered, given the family history. After all, grief and melancholia (as a major psychiatric mood disorder) do not only come together in the publications of Sigmund Freud and Melanie Klein.

Rose went through about six months of clinical psychotherapeutic treatment, at the end of which was day treatment. She was prescribed a combination of various antidepressants. Indeed, psychopharmaceuticals certainly played a major role in her treatment. They belong in the framework in that they create the enabling conditions for psychotherapy. The aim then is to get her to speak within an empathic and mirroring maternal environment. After all, her verbal and symbolic possibilities were minimal. She seemed stunned. She was very dependent but precise, meticulous, and inhibited in her actions, verging on compulsive perfectionism as if she didn't want to do anything wrong (anymore) because, in a way that was incomprehensible to her, she felt guilty that her father had left her life.

We only saw a turnaround when she started getting a bit angrier and 'naughty'. She got into conflicts with fellow patients and team members. She became cattier and a lot more frivolous in her appearance. While, at first, she 'couldn't be angry', her anger towards both her father and mother (who, after all, she felt each let her down in their own way) now become manifest and exert their 'right' in psychotherapy.

Rose started training and has been coming monthly for several years for supportive and consolidating follow-up. We can hardly call it a structural personality change, but grief work could be done. Also, her stunted psychosexual development came back on track. She was satisfied with these evolutions. The future will show if she wants more or to go further.

## Marina—Elegantly Found

This woman, in her late 20s, was referred because she said she was relapsing into old habits. She had previously been hospitalised several times at a PWGH service and other psychiatric hospitals because of anorexia and bulimia. 'I have problems with the physical.'

Marina has two half-brothers and four stepsisters. Her parents divorced when she was six, and she continued living with her mother. 'I wanted to be with mother to protect her.' Later, two new couples formed owing to previous games of partner swapping. Her father left for the southern sun with his new wife shortly after the divorce. She describes him as quiet, withdrawn, and closed off. He shows little sign of life and even less affective involvement. She has always craved his love and protection but never received them. Her mother is a blue-collar worker, described as a very naive woman who would also play dumb. According to Marina, she prattles, and, above all, her chatter is irrelevant. Marina can neither understand nor accept that her mother stayed with her new partner after what he did to her. This stepfather is described as a very aggressive and selfish man who controls her mother. He sexually abused and raped Marina almost daily between the ages of 6 and 15. It only stopped following her first period. Marina complained when one of her stepsisters was about to be abused. However, she was subsequently disowned and demonised by her mother's family. Marina has been quiet and shy since childhood, not wanting to bother anyone. She craves love, affection, and security and constantly feels scared and lonely. Since her adolescence, there has been a flight into polytoxicomania—cannabis, ecstacy, and cocaine. 'To not have to think, not have to feel anything.' She fled into a relationship with a man who was ten years older. She loved him desperately, but he left her for another woman. Since then, she has been in and out of hospital. 'No longer able and no longer wanting.' In the process, drug use has given way to cutting and eating problems, both of which she would have learned 'in psychiatry'.

Marina was in inpatient psychotherapy for over a year and has been coming for monthly outpatient treatment for about a decade since then. While an inpatient, she built a good, safe foundation with us. It also gave her clarity and insight into her post-traumatic issues as she was able to talk more about her sexual abuse, and her self-harming behaviour faded away. During her admission, she was courted by an elderly fellow patient who was married. Both parties were questioned about this several times, but they persisted and left.

Marina has neatly found peace and stability with her new partner. She feels safe because he cares for her materially and gives her livelihood security. He did prove to be an alcoholic and repeatedly takes a dim view of fidelity. This gives her good reason to reject his sexual advances and thus punish him for his misdeeds. She knows that she takes pleasure in making her husband pay. Nor is she alarmed by his increasing impotency problems—'what goes around comes around'. She has currently found a—for her—satisfactory balance. She now has a warm nest where—to her great satisfaction—sex is kept out.

## Freddy—All out of Nothing

This 30-something was referred from another clinical psychotherapy setting for the continuation of treatment because the predetermined three-month period there had expired. Previously, he had had several admissions to a regional general hospital. In the introductory interview, he complained of shyness: 'I don't know how to deal with people.' He tends to shut himself up and has a strong feeling of being unwanted, all the time and everywhere. He is desperate. 'It's been the same all my life.'

Spontaneously, Freddy starts talking about his mother, who told him he was not her son; that he was a fool; that it was even his fault that she was in pain during childbirth. She gave him many beatings and no opportunities. He was not allowed to study, not allowed to go to the youth movement, not allowed to invite friends over. He never knew his father. He did, however, see several men in the house.

Freddy is the youngest of four children, and they all have different fathers. Two of the eldest were taken away from home by the juvenile court because of abuse. He has not seen his mother for several years. 'She doesn't exist.' He was regularly beaten black and blue, and, when he was 12, she almost throttled him. This caused the world to collapse for him completely. 'I was nothing anymore.' He had to sleep on the streets and, from the age of 14, he had to go to work. He had to hand over everything and got neither clothes nor pocket money. She does not seek any contact with Freddy. Freddy received love and hugs only from a live-in uncle who, however, sexually abused him from adolescence onwards in exchange for clothes and toys.

He closed himself off, not feeling at home or comfortable anywhere. Socially, he was an outcast. 'I say things I don't want to say that hurt other people.' He plays guitar, draws, paints, and works with clay. He has studied English and German on his own. He can also spend hours working on computers and all kinds of appliances that he repairs. Machines, he says, are his best friends. 'I am completely self-made. I have a gift, but I am not allowed to use it.'

He finds himself among engineers who need to seek his advice in work situations. However, he does not rise higher because he lacks a degree, nor does he find formal recognition. He denounces the stupidity of others and the prevailing BTW (beer, tobacco, and wives) mentality. He had had two relationships so far that lasted about two years, in which he did everything for, and gave himself entirely to, his partner. However, they left him for another man and blamed him for disregarding them. He does not understand a thing.

Freddy has since been in clinical psychotherapy with us three times for several months. Each time, he left prematurely without saying goodbye to us or his fellow patients. Given the long distance and his lack of a car, he comes for low-frequency and irregular visits between and after admissions.

Before his initial admission, he lived as a hermit in a rural community where he was considered a village idiot. Even within the ward, the marginal position and isolation were repeated. He barely participated in the living-room and group events in the hospital unit. When he did attend, he bragged about his technical and creative ability and complained about an excessive and unstoppable creative urge that no one around him thanked him for.

While he looked down on therapists and fellow patients, there was a strong idealisation of me as an attending ward psychiatrist. In his eyes, I was Almighty God the Father and, thus, the only one with whom he could arrive at a meaningful conversation. He was keen to see his greatness and genius reflected in and through me. He was also initially—as was clear to everyone who had to deal with him—sitting on a time bomb of anger and hatred. However, he was hardly aware of any harm. The outside world was stupid and hostile; it did not understand him and recognised him even less. There was no self-reflection or self-criticism.

He only used the clinical psychotherapeutic mother environment to feed off our emotional care and attention. Throughout the three admissions, there was a remarkable evolution that took place mainly between the lines. Not only by telling his story himself and (daring to) show himself as increasingly small and vulnerable, but also by listening to the inner world of others, he became aware that he had a history of severe affective, material, and pedagogical neglect behind him, that he was full of abandonment rage and depression, that he had pulled himself out of the swamp by his hair by assuming a quasi-divine and self-satisfied status in which he seemed to need nothing and no one.

Freddy was, as it were, his creation ex nihilo, just as the Creator created Heaven and Earth out of nothing. He was an armed fortress where he could have retreated from a barren and hostile world. Reluctantly, through his music recordings, he left this bastion and was able to show the puny Freddy, who has always yearned for warmth, love, and recognition.

The latest consultations show that he has developed a good relationship with a staff member of the CPAS and that he volunteers there, repairing discarded appliances and items. He has also met some older volunteers there. He calls them comrades and occasionally goes for a beer with them, and they sometimes even drop in on him, unexpectedly and unannounced.

### Nadia—an Inexhaustible Source of Lead

Nadia is a woman in her early 30s who has undergone several long-term residential treatments. Each time, these were terminated because of persistent suicidal tendencies that had already led to several serious suicide attempts. It isn't easy to offer her sufficient security. She is the second of four children. Her mother is a housewife and is said to have a 'depressed core', according to Nadia. She only knows about food, clothes, and school and is always perceived by Nadia as not very warm. She was also very frugal and could enjoy nothing. While she was always at home and physically present, she was emotionally unavailable. 'Leave me alone; I am ironing.'

Her father was always outgoing and working. He was very career-oriented and status-sensitive, with excellent achievement drive. Nadia often felt laughed at by him. He labelled her in hurtful terms. Lately, as he has become more helpful and understanding, she has experienced him as borderline patronising. He reads all sorts of books on psychiatry and psychotherapy, and she feels he interferes too much in her intimate life. She has always felt distaste towards him.

Ever since she was a toddler, Nadia has been sad and tearful. She felt worthless and unimportant, especially compared with the younger sister who came after her. She bottled up a lot of pain, sadness, and anger but 'always carried on, no one ever knew'. She has a hard time living and is afraid of social contact. She has difficulty asking for help or revealing her problems. Anger is directed inward by her. She breaks down and self-destructs. Her initial self-harming occurred after a short, blunt reaction from her mother and following a storm of anger that rose within her, which she tried to calm down by herself.

In primary school, she feared failure, which she related to her father's teaching role. She felt she had to be perfect, had no girlfriends, was quiet, and retreated to the toilet during playtimes, waiting to go into a safer classroom situation under teacher supervision. During high school, she was socially inhibited, not daring to go out, act out, or be loose. She never had boyfriends—she was too shy. She never went out and was afraid of parties. She wore glasses, braces, and a corset because she had scoliosis. She was considered a 'nerd' and she felt like 'the hunchback of Notre Dame'.

Nadia studied at university 'to prove herself', especially to her father. She achieved excellent results there. During her student years, several one-night stands left her frustrated and abandoned. She has now been working in counselling for years. She is afraid of intimacy and nearness. She was in a relationship with a much older man, who was married and a father, for years. She kept this hidden from her parents all the time. He gave her courage and encouragement. He taught her to live and enjoy herself. Eventually, he left her for his wife, and she felt dumped. Both in her affair and her previous treatment, she felt rejected precisely when she dared to show her true, depressed face.

Nadia underwent over a year and a half of inpatient psychotherapy with us. She needed security, protection, and intensive care for a long time, given her persistent suicidal tendencies and attempts. She was joyless and dead, feeling sad and desperate, and she wandered around the ward like a zombie. She seemed at times like a death drive incarnate and had to contend continuously with a murderous inertia. The team regularly had to take over her vital functions, and the heart of our mother institute had to beat in place of her heart. She was in deep distress and had to be carried and nurtured by us like a baby. At the same time, there was something of a mute and subterranean passive resistance to whatever expectations were placed on her. For years, she had exhibited the following: pathological demand avoidance.

Nadia's bond with her parents also had many holes in it. She was stuck with a harsh, surly, harried, and disgruntled mother image that also haunted and inspected her from within. With her father, she had good contact only over the phone because she was annoyed by his smug and condescending paternalistic attitude.

Nadia had always upheld a false self and kept herself straight. Thanks to her intelligence and anxiously compulsive perfectionism, she had always excelled at school and university, so no one noticed anything wrong with her. Socially, moreover, she was very isolated. Her later work consumed all her available energy, and, after a day's work, she could only lie on her sofa or bed to recuperate until the following day.

Her whole edifice collapsed only after her lover abandoned her. She had known a period of true love with him, and only after she lost it all did the fundamental flaw of a lack of motherly love surface. The result was lethal melancholy.

In the course of her admission, she came into contact with abandonment, anger, and depression, as well as multiple narcissistic hurts. There swirled in her impulses of highly aggressive and spiteful feelings, especially towards her mother. Instead of exploding, she then lashed out at herself. Her poor bond and contact with her mother had set the tone for a generalised misanthropic disposition, where she shunned and even loathed fellow human beings. In particular, people who felt good and a fortiori smug aroused quasi-lethal envy in her. It was associated with a lot of resentment towards the father, who, after all, invariably disparaged or mocked her, resulting in a very poor self-image and low self-esteem.

Once the most profound depression had eased somewhat, she entered day treatment, and psychiatric help and support at home were organised, which, to this day, continue weekly. She has been coming to me weekly for psychotherapy for about five years and also goes to a behavioural therapist for coaching fortnightly. Her relationship with various therapists seems to be of great therapeutic importance. She feels supported, carried, and understood.

It took a lot of effort to identify the terrifying and oppressive mother image that was ensconced in her and free her from this demon's stranglehold. After years of struggling miserably against the law of inertia, she became a lot more agile in her demeanour and, not least, her tongue. She can sometimes be unusually sharp with it, at least in her feelings, because the outsider rarely feels the full charge of inner venom hidden in or behind her words.

Nadia also became well aware of the deficits in the mother–child relationship. She never felt positively affirmed or mirrored, and she could not go to her mother with other emotional needs and problems either. After all, her mother is blunt and succinctly straightforward. On the one hand, Nadia tries to comply with these demands, but, on the other hand, there is a little voice inside her that says no. The results are inertia, procrastination, time-wasting, and 'pulling and dragging' from morning to evening.

In recent years, she has had loose contact with three men: a somewhat unscrupulous adventurer who spends more time on exotic beaches than inland, an Asian with whom she has salacious chats, and an American with whom she communicates nightly about life and love. They are all 'virtual men', but this suits her well because it allows her to play without too much risk of (indeed serious) injury.

She has changed a lot in her appearance: she successfully put herself on a slimming diet, and dark or black clothing has given way to a brighter, more coquettish outfit, complemented by accessories that accentuate her femininity. A sometimes lively and enjoyable interaction ensues in the sessions, where wholehearted, out-loud laughter can be heard (including at one's problems and miseries).

Although she is terrified of falling back on to a gruelling treadmill of 'shoulds' and 'musts', she has agreed with her former employer to resume gainful extra hours under the progressive employment regime. A partner is not on her wish list for now. 'For that, I have become too fond of my hard-won freedom.'

## Petra—a Stepping Stone to Outpatient

This 20-year-old young woman was referred by the PWGH psychiatrist with whom she had previously been hospitalised a dozen times. Years before, she filed a formal legal complaint against her father for sexual assault and abuse. He was sentenced to effective jail time but was soon released.

Petra summarises her symptoms as flashbacks, nightmares, and self-destructive behaviour (hitting herself) against the background of a highly negative self-image. She is afraid to eat, which is related to all she has had to swallow (literally and figuratively) at the hands of her father. Her father is a construction worker and is described as highly aggressive, oppressive, and violent. He also drank excessively. He often walked around the house in women's clothes. She also saw him in women's underwear several times. Between the ages of 8 and 18, she was sadistically abused and raped by him almost daily. He also kept repeating that she was fat and stupid and that she stank. 'He grabbed me at my weakest moments.'

The patient's younger brother also received his share of blows (including with a hammer) from his father until he could 'defend himself in time'. Her mother is a housewife and never worked outside the home. She was said to be the complete opposite of the father, constantly letting herself be mistreated. Petra got on well with her. She has now given her a choice, prompting her to start divorce proceedings.

The patient said she did well emotionally in the first years of life. However, there were many fights and violence against the mother, in which she sustained several fractures. Petra can still see her walking around bleeding from a fork in her cheek that her father had stabbed her with. The father was falsely sweet and kind in public, but it was hell at home. Petra tried to zone out in her mind, hid everything away, and wept silently. All her feelings were switched off. She pretended that nothing touched her. Eventually, she told a friend a thing or two, which set the ball rolling.

Petra has been undergoing treatment with various orthopaedists, physical medicine specialists, and anaesthetists for years owing to diffuse, not always objectifiable, pain symptoms and is entirely disjointed, requiring surgical procedures, plastering, and other dressings. Although low-skilled, she possesses remarkable intelligence. She draws and paints and enjoys success with these. She had short-term relationships to get away from home, hoping to get out of her father's clutches. She has also been in a stable relationship for three years with a very gentle and caring man whom she is about to marry.

Petra was in clinical psychotherapy with us for only about three months. Despite her very severe traumatic experiences, she had strengths and talents, both verbal and artistic, symbolic, and sublimatory. Almost immediately, she began to see and experience me, the treating psychiatrist, as the father/perpetrator. Still, she was sensitive to interpreting these 'negative' transference reactions and immediately dealt with them constructively.

Excellent and smooth cooperation was quickly established with her psychotherapist. Partly given her difficulties with mobility, she promptly opted for intensive outpatient work with him. Ten years have passed since then. After her discharge, she never came to see me again. Not long ago, however, I received an invitation to an exhibition in which she was participating. It came with a card thanking me and saying: 'Still with [...] in psychotherapy. It's on the right track, but there's still some way to go.'

## Arnold—the Perfect Wave

Arnold is a 40-something referred by his GP for outpatient psychotherapy. He has been coming weekly for about eight years now. He has a remarkable physical appearance: he dresses entirely in black, in winter and summer. The shape of his head is also unusual and, therefore, conspicuous. He has a highly elongated face and almost unnaturally long arms and legs, making him seem almost alien.

Here are his opening words:

> In the long run, the thing is that I have always struggled and never really functioned well in social groups, never accepted into them. I have no trouble with rules or with maintaining minimal social contact. However, I have always put things off regarding more intimate relationships. One important thing that has triggered a whole new line is that I started feeling more for a female colleague ten years ago. I realise it is fundamental, and my story fits my early teenage years. If I told people that, they would say: how old are you anyway? I had been noticing that colleague for a while, and then I got her attention, and that's when I started dissecting the situation and immediately saw a lot of possibilities of what things could mean. In that first moment, I panicked a bit. Afterwards, I tried to make tentative contact. Then I had these feelings for her. I asked to go for a drink, and we did. And then I had the constant doubt: is that a positive response from her, or is it just out of politeness? Doubt. When I say that, it can sound a bit childish. I feel less justified in my thinking and

my feelings. When we had gone for a drink, I thought the conclusion was that she did not want further contact. That was ten years ago. Then there was a period when I thought my colleagues were giving all kinds of signals, trying to make things clear to me, for example, by dropping her name significantly. I also had all kinds of scenarios about what I should do. Scenarios to make contact. Working in a pleasant atmosphere, I approached colleagues. They knew nothing about it. In the end, I then approached a colleague who was a psychologist by training and who, after conversations, concluded that seeing signals from others was a problem and that I was forming theories on it that fitted into my stall ... I want to add that I don't have difficulties interpreting someone, but I am much more sensitive to how someone else thinks and feels. So it's not that I have a hard time empathising with someone. From the conversations with that psychologically trained colleague, it further emerged that I was not allowed to pay so much attention to those signals that may or may not exist. Also, maybe I was too motivated to do something for that woman, but then I backed off to the next step. Later, I sent an extensive e-mail to her, to which she informed me not to push for a relationship especially because we were colleagues at work ... I realised that I could not entirely trust my interpretations, but that did not solve my problem of loneliness.

Arnold is the eldest of four sons. His father is a retired civil servant, and his mother is a housewife. They divorced about a decade before. There have always been arguments and scenes between his parents. Unlike his younger brothers (because his parents both left work later), Arnold was raised by the maternal grandparents. His grandfather is described as a quiet and good-natured man. He was somewhat overprotective. The father is also described as a reasonable and calm man with whom he could communicate well.

The grandmother and mother are both highly unreasonable in his eyes. They make noise for no reason, they nitpick at trifles, and react to their surroundings when they are not feeling well mentally or physically. Their hyper-emotional 'hysterics' terrorise their family members. He attributes the fact that he is sensitive to accusations and constantly afraid of doing wrong to their influence. It will later be revealed that the mother is said to have had several psychiatric admissions and attempted suicide several times.

Arnold feels anxious, insecure, misunderstood, and maltreated. He has long thought things would work out if he followed the rules, but things don't work out because there are no rules. He constantly tried to be accepted and loved but kept feeling abandoned and rejected. Through his account, there was love, but that could suddenly turn around because of any fact or detail. He had little freedom of movement as both the grandmother and mother were prudes. Everything had to be in perfect order. You were almost afraid to move.

I always knew it was purely their fault and responsibility. I never felt guilty. All the family recognised that. My mother and grandmother's states were considered a kind of natural phenomenon, a kind of earthquake. There was nothing they could do about it. They were nervous. We were within our rights.

It further appears that, with his grandparents, he was given few boundaries and many toys. They constantly kept him inside. He was neither encouraged to be, nor made, self-reliant. Until the age of 15, he never walked the streets alone. He was always accompanied by his grandfather, who otherwise constantly engaged with him and talked to him about all kinds of 'life wisdom'. However, he was never given a goal by him. All that mattered was earning a living, health, and other 'trivial things'. 'Just make sure your head is not above the parapet', he scornfully says.

He was a good student but consistently especially strong on concepts. He was always very slow, for example, in tests or exams. 'I think too much and too far before I start answering.' He obtained a high school diploma and has worked permanently as a civil servant in Brussels for many years. He is one of those countless commuters who commute to the capital in a state between sleep and waking.

After much thought and mulling on trains and platforms, he cautiously nods a greeting to women who address him in any way. He tries to gauge from their facial expressions and body language whether and to what extent they are open to him. At work, he zooms in on everyday occurrences and interactions in the canteen, in the break room, or at the photocopier. After much preliminary thinking, he tries to trace or provoke something emotionally meaningful.

From the first interviews, I thought of a fundamentally dated encounter with his mother/the woman. I associated his story with the film *Contact*, in which Jodie Foster uses a giant telescope to search for extraterrestrial life. He repeatedly talked about problems that seemed to have existed for as long as he could remember, thus dating back to his primaeval or prehistoric days. It was then about the sandpit and kindergarten, where he played independently and failed to connect with other little kids.

In primary school, a girl had a crush on him. At one point, she drew a dinosaur that he had brought to class and gave him the drawing as a gift. He rejected this gesture of love and even criticised her drawing. I understood it as a painfully ill-fated *close encounter* where a passive-active reversal occurred, and he acted, exceptionally, as the rejecter rather than the rejected.

In adolescence, he went to the cinema for the first time. It was a revelation. Over the years, he developed cinephile interests, taste, and sensibility. He brought to consultations about a hundred stills from feature films, which he commented on extensively and with stunning pertinence in the sessions. Note that the (im)possibility of contact and rapprochement was a thematic constant.

In his young adulthood, he discovered heavy metal music, and he occasionally attended concerts where he joined the headbanging crowd. I learn that his black clothes have more to do with this scene than with the French existentialists associated with *Les Temps Modernes*. He has retained a childhood friend here and there from his teenage years, but contacts between them have died out one by one. Since his amorous adventure is mentioned, he makes more of an effort to 'get out there'. He attends lectures and talks of a general cultural but mainly philosophical nature, and, judging by the names and references he drops here and there, he is pretty in tune with even the most recent developments in the field. Once in a while, he goes on a city trip with his brother. The description of these excursions is apt: 'We stay in a kind of bubble, have contact with nothing or nobody. It is like walking on a treadmill, and various cityscapes pass as if on a screen'.

Arnold's narrative is constant in form. It is consistently very rational, intellectualising, and abstract. He produces theoretical views and expectations about love and married life. Again, the metaphor of extraterrestrial intelligence comes to mind. Even when all the finer points of (inter)human life are mapped out, incurable stunting will undoubtedly be involved in practice. After all, it has to do with initial (and early childhood) socialisation, after which one can hardly ever develop as a true 'natural' in even the most mundane matters.

Given that the problems are so deep, I suggested admission for inpatient psychotherapy at first and also later. There are multiple reasons why I recommended and advocated this. First, it provides an environment in which a profound regression is possible. You can go back to the start, as it were, and recalibrate psychosocial and psychosexual development. Treatment is intensive, and the more resources you invest (including human), the faster (or less slowly) the psychotherapeutic process succeeds. Virtually all activities occur in small or large groups, making social problems visible, workable, and discussable, and involving interactive learning. Last but not least, the therapy programme contains many expressive activities (such as visual work, dance and music therapy) that also include preverbal media of communication and developmental assistance. They then draw on the same analogue repertoire available to mammals and the early childhood environmental mother.

Between dream and deed, laws stand in the way, and practical objections. Arnold could not opt for this treatment (and the long-term medical work incapacity it implied). As a rule, when people are physically damaged, they opt to have a major surgical procedure, even if this involves risks and a longer or shorter rehabilitation. When it comes to psychological suffering, taking such a step and making such a decision is usually a lot less obvious.

Over the years, Arnold developed a lot of imagery for his problems. Right from introductory talks, he talked about his 'skin hunger'. It scared people and invariably made them think he wanted 'more'. He denied this in words, but, on the other hand, eye contact or a smile was enough to trigger fantasies about a relationship's ups and downs, the dos and don'ts.

The term 'skin hunger' naturally confirmed my hypothesis about the origin of the problem. It seemed rooted in that first stage of life where we still know 'skin-ache', when skin hunger is insufficiently satisfied. To unearth this primal layer, I quoted a verse by the Flemish modernist poet Paul van Ostaijen, 'I want to be naked and start', which Arnold returned to many times in psychotherapy.

In time, he also talked about his lion suit. He had concluded that something about his 'pack' apparently frightened fellow humans or made them recoil. In the course of psychotherapy, a lot of anger and resentment appeared alongside sadness. Arnold himself (rightly, in my view) believes he has an open and broad-minded mind. He has a lot of positive acceptance towards (even narrow-minded or civil) fellow human beings. On the other hand, he notes that he has to meet relatively narrow and limited expectations from others. Is there something about his appearance that does not please others? I, at one point, suggested the thought experiment of what would happen should he show up in a crayon suit from now on. There was some hilarity, and it gradually became more common for us to laugh together at this or that statement.

I do not rule out that elements of an autism spectrum disorder would be retained if he was subjected to psychodiagnostic testing. In many patients, such recognition means identifying the grain of sand that makes the social engine turn square. Invisible impairment can be more constructively integrated (but not removed), and necessary lifestyle adjustments can be introduced (with or without additional professional help). Considering that Arnold was working and could broadly hold his own quite well, I feared the disadvantages of needless reification. By labelling, one risks producing a cap on meaning, which stops a process of increasing subjectification.

Two other comparisons surfaced in his story. Early in psychotherapy, he compared his problem to a patient who did not even manage to get through to the waiting room. The door does not open for him. The symbolic implications of this fateful disposition are sufficiently clear. Did he fear he could not reach me (as a mother and wife)?

After several years of therapy, he introduced a new metaphor. He talked about a surfer standing on the beach with his board under his arm, waiting for the right wave. The comparison is apt. In most cases, it is (thankfully) love between the mother and her infant at first sight. If this is not the case, a first infatuation runs aground, and a hitch/snag can also develop in other (first) contacts and/or infatuations, with more or less catastrophic consequences.

The first bond with the mother forms through successive (micro)moments of encounter strung together like a chain and based on a playful interaction inimitable to others. This is partly owing to that particular state of mind in which a mother 'in shape' finds herself during the first period after childbirth.

All indications are that Arnold was deprived of this simultaneously average and exceptional experience. It is also quite possible that both mother and grandmother themselves displayed elements of autism spectrum disorder.

Arnold remains fruitlessly searching for a *Close Encounter*, with a nod to Steven Spielberg's feature film, which is not of the third but of the *first kind*.

## Berthe—Too Young and Too Old

Berthe is a 30-year-old young woman who was hospitalised in a juvenile psychiatric setting during her adolescence. Since then, she has been in continuous outpatient care with two women: a psychiatrist and a psychologist. This has kept her 'straight' and allowed her to pursue higher studies and obtain professional work, but, apart from that, her life is at a dead end. As a single person, she lives a very isolated and poor existence. She works in the care sector and tries ('like a Duracell rabbit') to live up to everyone's expectations, but, in the evenings, she is exhausted and worn out and hardly gets to live her own (private) life.

Berthe's parents ran a bakery, and both died. Her father died of a heart attack about two years earlier. He is described as a somewhat absent figure with alcohol problems who was under the thumb of his mother and did not care much for the children. Everything had to go forwards, and you were not allowed to 'moan'. He could, however, be smooth and pleasant in his dealings and even occasionally be 'witty'.

However, Berthe never felt completely safe and at ease with her father. She has memories of transgressive behaviour and sexual remarks/talk by her father. She did not feel seen by him but (wrongly—because in a perverse way) watched by him. She caught her parents or her father watching porn films on several occasions. She was also occasionally an ear witness to her parents' lovemaking, which greatly confused and frightened her. She had nightmares from her primary school days in which both her father and mother sexually harassed her. She, on the other hand, is convinced that she was never actually sexually abused or harassed. However, she does retain a profound aversion to anything to do with sexuality as a result of all this, she says.

Berthe is the youngest of three daughters. The older two were bright and promising students who, in her eyes, received more love and attention because her parents were only interested in school achievements and social prestige. She has always felt different and unwanted, as well as the fifth wheel on the cart. She constantly went out of her way to please her mother, for instance, by being very accommodating or surprising her with all kinds of self-made presents that invariably ended up in the bin.

She never felt valued or loved by her mother but, on the contrary, hurt and rejected. She recalls wandering around the house, often searching for her footing and (also literal) reflection. For instance, she sometimes stood for hours in front of the mirror in the parental bedroom. After all, she struggled to hold herself together.

Her mother died of a brain tumour about ten years earlier. Berthe was very affected by her physical deterioration. She died at home, and Berthe was expected to provide care even in its most intimate aspects. She retains many grim images and painful memories from this time, especially since she had never had a close relationship with her mother. There were always many discussions and misunderstandings. 'Mum was always angry.' 'I couldn't do anything right for her.'

From childhood, Berthe was quiet, well-behaved, withdrawn, and shy. 'I was never allowed to be weak/sick.' Instead of sending SOS messages, she pasted them behind the wallpaper. If you were on a desert island, you would throw your 'message in a bottle' into the sea. She says she was always a wallflower during her adolescence. Consequently, she has no relational or sexual experience whatsoever. She by no means lacks physical attraction, but she says she feels far too scared and insecure. Besides, she has little connection with anything or anyone. She is orphaned and neglected, overflowing with abandonment rage and depression, and is constantly immersed in re-experiences in the 'haunted house' that was the parental home.

We were all once number one in everyday events and were at the centre of attention and interest 24/7. This first period of life provides a basis for a self (value) that cannot be found anywhere else to that extent. Berthe felt like she had been untethered all her life, not having found anything to hold on to, such as understanding and especially positive acceptance and mirroring. She was full of, and still surrounded by, a past in which she was lost in her childhood home, watching from her room as her parents sat cosily in the kitchen, eating and chatting with her two older sisters while she sat alone and in exile, moping in her room.

How often did she sit and watch the neighbours through the window, trying to absorb from afar the sense of home and family that seemed to prevail there? She had several white rabbits as pets and playmates, but each time they ended mercilessly in the cooking pot and on the plate. She took refuge in daydreams, fairy tales, and fantasy stories and longed for the proverbial prince on a white horse who would come and free her from her plight of isolation sooner or later.

Berthe looked up to her female therapists for many years. They were surrogate mothers for whose support and appreciation she tried to make progress (at least at the study and social level). Eventually, however, she collapsed from too many needs too long unmet. She was in inpatient psychotherapy with us for several years and has been attending as an outpatient twice a week for two years now. She was very fragile and clingy throughout most of her admission, constantly seeking reassuring closeness and care from the nursing team. A pathological—that is, symptomatic—dependence developed, especially towards her female individual psychiatric nurse.

Berthe latched on to her from the first to the last minute of her presence on the ward and (without exaggeration) chased her into the toilets. There was an anxious insistence on expressions of love. Did she have a place in her individual nurse's heart? Was she special? Did this nurse have warm feelings for her? For a long time, Berthe 'used' the admission situation to regain the love, care, and attention she had missed as a child.

Thanks to sustained mentalising development aid and interpretation, she could 'place' these deficits more and leave them somewhat behind. It was as if she did not want to grow but wanted to be small (again) and be reborn in or on the lap of our ward. In the absence of parents, given the mocking and condescending attitude of her older sisters, and in the absence of a circle of family or friends, support from her home environment was nil. She, therefore, felt that her whole life depended entirely on us.

It took quite a lot of socialising support to get her into day treatment and, eventually, out on discharge: psychiatric help at home, voluntary work, and job coaching. In her own words, Berthe built basic security and a more positive and stable sense of self with us. She is looking for paid work she could still take up because caring for older people and having a job filled with 'piss and poop' is something she no longer sees fit to do.

Now that she is in outpatient psychotherapy, her sexual problems have come to the fore. She is trying dating and has been to bed with several men several times. She then suffers from vaginismus to an extreme degree. Of her own accord, she has started seeking help from a sexologist, but it is a fruitless mess, with various sex toys and attachments. Would she hire a gigolo? Let herself be taken by the first of the best to break the 'roadblock'? Meanwhile, she brings up in detail her revenge in the bikini region.

In her mid-30s, she feels simultaneously too young and too old. She is too young because she still needs care and is not ready to take on basic tasks and responsibilities. She is too old to experience puberty and adolescence, to explore amorously and erotically and to take first steps (only now) sexually. She is angry because everyone expected her to tag along without ensuring that she could develop sufficiently psychosocially and sexually.

## Werner—Stuttering between Poacher and Forester

His treating psychiatrist referred this 40-something because of long-standing depressive symptoms that have made him medically unable to work for some time.

Werner is the eldest of three children. He has two younger sisters with whom he has little contact. The mother is described as depressed. For a long time, Werner had a close relationship with her. He was her support and advocate. As a boy, he saw her washing herself in a tub in the bedroom several times—a nude scene that made him feel very uncomfortable. His mother also shared her bedtime and other secrets with him. Things never really worked between his parents. They have lived under the same roof as if divorced for years.

Werner has suffered with a stutter since he was about ten years old and was bullied and mocked a lot for this. He has been sexually aware since primary school. He is seduced by the erotic pictures to be seen at the entrance of a local cinema and, from early puberty, he has masturbated daily. His mother repeatedly confronted him with the marks ('dirt') this left, which made him feel very embarrassed and angry. There was also an incident where the mother showed his dirty pants to his father on his return home after an accidental moment of incontinence. The pain, anger, humiliation, and powerlessness remain palpable after all these years when he recounts it. 'It was suddenly two against one.'

Werner continued to live at home until he was 30. He moved out then, but his mother continued to do his laundry even after that. Indeed, he has great difficulty caring for himself and maintaining a minimum of order and cleanliness. His father is described as sullen, moody, and introverted. Werner has hardly any contact with him. In any case, he missed out on a lot of empathy and companionship because of his father. However, he shares great social engagement with his father. His father was in the trade union, and, at home, there was often talk about the class struggle and the exploitation of 'the little man'.

After taking a classical humanities degree, Werner dreamed of studying higher art at the academy. Failing the entrance exam was a significant frustration. He was advised to retake it, as he reportedly did not lack talent, but he was so disappointed and aggrieved that he 'refused' to make a second attempt. He then went on a pilgrimage, on foot, for several weeks, and this was the beginning of lingering depressive symptoms.

Werner did have higher qualifications in counselling and had already had several jobs in the care sector. However, he repeatedly struggled with laws, rules, and authority, to which, gritting his teeth, he submitted but, sooner or later, he clashed with or resented them and quit. With regard to relationships, in his best years (in retrospect, for far too long), he was in a relationship with a married woman. He always just waited for her. When she got pregnant by him, she aborted the baby and left him for good. This broke him even more. At the time of admission, he was in a living-apart-together relationship with a divorced woman.

Werner was in (day) clinical psychotherapy for about three years, with interruptions of several months. Since then, he has been coming for weekly face-to-face psychotherapy. Some of his difficulties and sensitivities were acted out during the admission. He repeatedly sought maternal concern and 'empathy', but, in our safe and protective environment, he soon found himself in the mode of criticising and rebelling against departmental operations and rules. He then appeared as a rebel leader who spoke up and challenged managers in group meetings. He did a lot of sports and was very competitive and combative. He enjoyed the attention of fellow female patients, and, on several occasions, there were crushes on much younger women, including some in the team.

Phasing out day therapy and certainly trying to get him back to work or employment in the outside world invariably met with a lot of resistance. He worked for periods but, each time, he quickly developed depressive symptoms. On closer inspection, this 'depression' was more about regressive tendencies in which he appealed for maternal care and support as well as displaying passive-aggressive resistance to any form of power or authority. At one point, it came up that he gave his father's state the finger, albeit wrapped in a certificate for being medically unfit for work.

Not only did he experience difficulty accepting others' authority, but he also found great difficulty exercising authority over others. In the course of his psychotherapy, he started writing poetry, which he sent to me and, with an anxious heart, had me read. He knew that I, too, had written some occasionally, and he was terrified of being reprimanded by me for these literary attempts. At some point, he started wearing a hat and was also very wary of how his father would react. Apart from a dry remark about the difference between a 'John' with a cap and a John with a hat, he—to his surprise—got off lightly (because he was not punished).

Werner loves dogs. They are his best and most loyal friends. However, they often cause vibrations in the sensitive string of master–servant relationships. Who is the boss over whom? Do they have to be on a leash, or can they roam freely in nature? On his long forest walks, he fears being reprimanded by foresters but, on the other hand, has a lot of vicarious pleasure in letting his dogs roam freely.

He shows himself to women mainly as a wolf in sheep's clothing, but he lets his lustful eye fall on many a 'goat'/girl. He likes to feel mighty and lord and master in sexual situations but is afraid of falling into a woman's clutches. He often gets stuck halfway in his advances. The engine of his love life splutters. He feels violent urges churning but is afraid of losing control to them. He also fears clashing with rivals or being kept under the thumb of Mother-the-Wife.

When he came knocking for admission for the umpteenth time after a period of outpatient therapy, we deliberately kept the hospitalisation very short that time. Angry at this rejection, he looked for another psychotherapist closer to him and, for a while, came to me only monthly for psychiatric and process counselling. He said he needed support and coaching more than further digging into his history.

However, following new love upsets, he resumed psychotherapy with me a few months later. Only now are his mother and father both, simultaneously, starting to come into the picture. For the first time, he sees connections between his desire to shine on stage or in a woman's lap and his fear that she will be 'in his trousers' and/or arouse a father's scorn and wrath. Indeed, he catches himself being attracted to women 'on the other side of the bar' every time. He flirts with them, fantasises about them, and stays 'fixated' on them for (far) too long and against his better judgement.

By now, we agree on *what* habitually continues to falter or stutter. Although the stuttering has now been entirely absent for many years, we have never analysed this symptom in detail. Like most other symptoms, it is only the tip of the iceberg and disappears when enough has melted underwater.

## Gaston—out of the Wolfpack

This 40-something was referred because of lingering depressive symptoms for which there have already been three admissions to PWGH services. He has been consulting with various psychiatrists and psychologists since young adulthood, but all this has not helped him much. 'I was always pushed from home to study and work and see where I am now', he says, full of resentment and bitterness.

Gaston is the middle of three children. His younger brother was born with multiple disabilities and has always grabbed a lot of care and attention from his parents. Gaston, too, has always been protective and cares for him. He describes his parents as tough businesspeople with little room for his little pains. His mother comes from a family of entrepreneurs and bears the marks of that. She never saw much emotion.

The father is described as a selfish *bon vivant* who cares little for the children and other domestic concerns. He is portrayed as a macho 'male chauvinist'. From childhood, Gaston felt belittled and castigated by hurtful remarks made by his father. This made him insecure and timid, feeling 'psychologically impotent'. He was also literally always worried about the shape and size of his penis and had great doubts as an adolescent but could not go to anyone with this. There were great feelings of inferiority towards peers. He was reserved to downright avoidant where the opposite sex was concerned.

He threw himself into studies and odd jobs early to compensate. His father also called on Gaston's unpaid hand- and footwork on occasion. 'He is a real money-grubber.' To make matters worse, he suffered a poorly treated torsion of his testicles around the age of 18, requiring unilateral castration. He has a testicular prosthesis and has since feared infertility or the loss of the remaining testicle, in addition to impotence.

Having earned two bachelor's degrees, he has always worked hard. In recent years, however, he has been 'broken' by various health problems. As a result of bankruptcy, he has been unemployed for two years and is struggling to make ends meet. What weighs most heavily is that he has neither a partner nor children. 'I made the wrong choices.'

Gaston was hospitalised for about six months and, after that, came for outpatient treatment for another two years or so. He was literally and figuratively filled with anger, and his psychotherapy was initially a long-drawn-out tirade against his parents, by whom he felt short-changed, mistreated, and abandoned. Only after all this explosive material had been sufficiently discharged did he begin to see his parents as people of flesh and blood. People who had their qualities and flaws and whose lack of understanding was based more on misunderstanding than malice.

He compared himself to Shakespeare's Richard III, who was furious with the world, life, and the human race because of a congenital deformity.

A crucial therapeutic point was that I tuned into his misery empathically, in a sustained manner. Only when he had found sufficient understanding and recognition could he show himself as softer, more vulnerable. He dared, for instance, to recount in detail his painful experiences in the bedroom. He figuratively dropped his trousers and built enough security and trust to face his deep-seated fear of a blunt father.

A major issue that remained present throughout therapy concerned finances. It was often about the duration of our sessions and my fee. Several times, he didn't show up for our appointment. However, I talked to him about fees for missed appointments without even charging them. Thanks to this balancing act, his fears that I would exploit him like his father and that I was a fat, heartless capitalist could be discussed.

It was undisputable that his unjustified absences were the symbolic equivalent of a raised middle finger. He was extremely grateful that I did not make him pay for such rebellion but merely tried to acknowledge and name the feelings and sensitivities underlying it. When he found new work and our schedules no longer fitted, he stopped therapy.

## Yolande—the Dark Side of the Moon

Yolande was in her late 20s when she was hospitalised owing to major depression and suicidal tendencies. This wasn't her first time receiving psychiatric care; she had previously been admitted several times to PWGH services, including after a severe incident where she stabbed herself in the abdomen with a meat cleaver after being rejected by someone she loved.

She is the youngest of three daughters and outwardly appeared to have no major issues. Her father, a strict and formal man, had built a successful corporate career but was largely uninvolved in raising his children. According to Yolande, he was proper and sensitive but struggled to discuss emotional matters. On the other hand, her mother was a tender-hearted woman with little emotional understanding and high expectations about status and appearances.

Yolande was obedient and shy from childhood, always striving to meet her mother's expectations. However, she never felt comfortable in the feminine role imposed upon her. She often felt more like a boy than a girl, but was constantly being dressed up like a princess for her mother. She felt she was treated like a doll. While her friends played with Barbies, Yolande preferred playing with the boys in the neighbourhood. She reluctantly took ballet lessons at her mother's insistence, though she would have preferred judo. Throughout high school, she had few friends and described herself as a know-it-all and an overachiever. She didn't feel she experienced typical puberty, though she did develop crushes on several teachers and fantasised about being their sweetheart.

Yolande excelled in higher education, consistently achieving top marks and becoming the perpetual top student. However, her problems began at university, where she struggled with a profound identity crisis. She didn't know who she was or what she wanted, and she began questioning her sexual identity. During her successful studies, she developed intense crushes on several women, which were mostly unreciprocated. Her feelings became so obsessive that one woman even filed a complaint against her for stalking. This period was marked by intense inner turmoil and confusion.

Yolande spent about two years in clinical psychotherapy, including day therapy. From the beginning, her treatment focused on what was understood as a false self problem: she had spent her life trying to meet her mother's expectations without feeling truly seen or recognised for who she was. There was a 'dark side of the moon' within her—an unexpressed, hidden part of herself full of abandonment, rage, and depression. These feelings had been repressed and never fully processed or integrated. This understanding provided a framework for her therapy, offering a container for the various emerging emotions and sensitivities.

As expected, Yolande developed a close relationship with the ward—or environment mother—and her female psychotherapist, seeking to satisfy many unmet emotional needs. However, this attachment carried the risk of boundary violations, as her feelings of love and hate intertwined in a volatile mix—a Molotov cocktail of love and hate. It required her therapist to walk a fine line between expressing empathy and setting appropriate boundaries.

During treatment, Yolande invented a new symptom. She took up intensive sports and, over time, took up cycling, especially mountain biking. There was a lot of raw and unrefined temper in her that she used as fuel for motoric release. She was very concerned with her physical fitness and appearance and enjoyed a both androgynous and eternally youthful appearance. In one of her dreams, she had the outline of a polished penis.

On a relational level, there was simultaneously a relationship with a fellow cyclist who, like her, showed a somewhat fluid gender identity as he was bisexual by orientation. He was a true soulmate or other-equal with whom she got to experience a lot of support and affirmation on good and bad days. On the other hand, there was a somewhat older, married female colleague at work with whom she officially went out and travelled as a close friend, but with whom she clandestinely maintained an erotic and romantic affair with all the excitement, thrills, and naughty pleasures that this entailed.

With her high school qualifications and fragile emotional state, finding a proper job was not easy. In several workplaces, she lost herself in an excessive desire to perform. Long hours and working days were accompanied by procrastination and inefficiency that, over time, could be understood as ambivalence towards the expectations of (maternal) superiors. She eventually joined a non-governmental organisation with a flexible working arrangement that allowed her the necessary freedom of movement for sports. After about five years of weekly outpatient psychotherapy, she chose to phase out monthly follow-up sessions, which she stopped after a year, satisfied with the professional and relational balances achieved.

# Chapter 5

# Modus Operandi

Many years ago, I received permission from more than 100 (former) patients to devote a case study to their problems. See below for the informed consent I sent them to avoid wasting precious consultation time. Some of them asked to read their section before publication. Naturally, this was done. Their main concern was whether anonymity would be sufficiently guaranteed. Here and there, they commented on the content—for instance, by clarifying or elaborating on specific details.

I kept no more than 77 cases in this book. They provide a sufficiently truthful sample of a psychotherapeutic practice.

I thank those involved for their permission to publish and the trust this demonstrates.

Dear _____,

Subject: informed consent/written consent.

I want to ask you a somewhat unusual question. As part of the Current Psychoanalytics series www.psychoanalytischactueel.eu, I am preparing a book on psychoanalysis and psychiatry. Taking 100 case studies from a practice of inpatient and outpatient psychotherapy as my starting point for over 20 years, I will elucidate several aspects of contemporary theory and practice for a professional readership. I, at this moment, request permission to use clinical data from your psychological and psychiatric problems for a case report. According to the usual deontological rules for scientific publication, your data will be anonymous. Of course, if you wish, you may formulate questions, reservations or comments either via e-mail or in a personal contact. Sign this letter with 'for agreement' for your informed consent.

Sincerely,

Dr Kinet

www.markkinet.be

DOI: 10.4324/9781003490609-5